THERAPEUTIC SOLUTIONS FOR COVID

THE MEDICINE AND DRUGS TO TREAT CORONAVIRUS

Susan Su

Copyright © 2023 *Susan Su*

All Rights Reserved

CONTENTS

PREFACE

Ever since 2019, I have been collecting newspaper and magazine, internet articles, academic papers on various therapeutic solutions for COVID-19. As the world battle coronavirus for three years, the therapeutic solution is proved to be absolutely necessary and crucial.

This book summarizes various medicine treatment as therapeutic solution for COVID-19 in different stage of infection to prevent from coronavirus infection and its progression in human body. Those include the CDC and World Health Organization approved ones, clinical trial proved ones as well as proved effective home treatment methods.

The knowledge of the book is based on scientific report, authority website, published academic journal papers. They are presented intuitively in easy to understand language for everyone to read.

DISCLAIMER

Unless cited the source and referred to the original website and reference, the points in the book otherwise represent the author's own opinion and scientific view. The book is mainly for education and knowledge purpose. All questions and health issues should be referred to your healthcare specialist.

CHAPTER 1. INTRODUCTON

-THE PANDEMIC TODAY

Since the original coronavirus outbreak in December 2019, the arrival of New Year 2023 marks the full three years of the world battle the then, and now still "novel" coronavirus--COVID-19. What does the new year of pandemic mean to us? The original coronavirus RNA muted with human being body cell to produce many muted new virus, now with more human cell's RNA, become less "alien" to human body. Therefore, they did not cause such a dramatic immune system reaction as the original ones. People who catch the virus now react with more like some kind of flu virus symptom. The symptom become less severe even though they become more infectious.

So what does the New Year of 2023 have to bring? -- Hopefully Big Good News--The world will get over with COVID. To be accurately, COVID will be all over the world; almost everyone will get it; then get over with it; same as the 1918 Spanish Flu mysteriously disappeared by itself after two or three years. They did not disappear, they just became less harmful and everyone got it and got over with it. As many people in the community catch the virus and get over with it, enough people in the population are immune to an infectious disease. The disease is then unlikely to spread from person to person. This is known as 'community immunity' (also referred to as 'herd immunity'). How eventually the pandemic come to the full stop. As so many people catch COVID, the therapeutic treatment, what medicines to take when one catches COVID become crucially important.

Even with various vaccination, the new coronavirus string, such as Omicron, still can invade since the vaccine was based on a previous coronavirus RNA sequence. For example, there are four types of infections from mosquito bites: A, B, C, D. If one gets type A infection, the antibody generated will only protect him/her from reinfection by type A, not the other types of B, or C, or D. Also if one caught type B after type A infection, the symptom will be even more severe than not catching type A at all. Does this principle apply to various coronavirus variants infection? In the author's opinion, theoretically it shall apply straightforward--vaccine has to base on the RNA of same string of various. But without clinical data to verify, the author can't see very much about the vaccine while the authority says "Some people will experience mild to moderate side effects after being vaccinated against COVID-19. This is a normal sign that the body is developing protection". Clinical data had proved that the mosquito bite principles apply to monoclonal antibody therapies. For example, monoclonal antibodies bamlanivimab/etesevimab and casirivimab/imdevimab had been proved by clinical evidence that they were cloned/copied from an earlier various strings, only working effectively for these string infection. They won't work for the newly muted strings, such as Omicron. For the new string, with the old antibody generated, the symptoms were clinically proved to become worse. In order for a monoclonal antibody to treat and work for newly mated string such as Omicron, they need to be cloned/copied from the antibody produced by one infected by Omicron.

But it is a well-known and proved truth, that even though one received vaccine, he or she can still become infected by another newly muted coronavirus string. With the emergence of the antigenically distinct variants of concern, either natural immunity or first-generation vaccine-induced immunity has failed to prevent transmission effectively. Since April 2022, BA. 2.12. 1, BA. 4, and BA. 5 subvariants of the omicron (B. 1.1. 529) have been spreading globally with increased viral fitness and transmissibility. Omicron

BA.5 subvariant is currently the predominant COVID-19 threat worldwide.

It is estimated that a new variant string comes every three months. With so many muted coronavirus variants, the therapeutic solution become even more important. As the world battle COVID for over three years, we now know more about the virus and have several medicine treatments. Some are approved by the World Health Organization (WHO) and CDC. Some are sold by private company; some are simple at- home treatment methods. The following chapters describe these therapeutic solutions.

CHAPTER 2. BACKGROUND INFORMATION

2.1 General Information on COVID-19

Infectious diseases prevalent in humans and animals are caused by pathogens that once emerged from other animal hosts. In addition to these established infections, new infectious diseases periodically emerge. In extreme cases, they may cause pandemics such as COVID-19, and in other cases, dead-end infections or smaller epidemics result.

In late December 2019, a novel coronavirus was identified in China (Wuhan) causing severe respiratory disease including pneumonia. On February 11, 2020, the Coronavirus Study Group of the International Committee on Taxonomy of Viruses issued a statement announcing an official designation for the novel virus: severe acute respiratory syndrome coronavirus 2 (SARS-CoV-2). The respiratory illness caused by SARS-CoV-2 was termed COVID-19 by the World Health Organization (WHO), the acronym derived from "coronavirus disease 2019". The name was chosen to avoid stigmatizing the virus's origins in terms of populations, geography, or animal associations.

The World Health Organization (WHO) advised the following language associated with the virus. "The coronavirus disease 2019 (COVID-19) is a communicable respiratory disease caused by a new strain of coronavirus that causes illness in humans. Coronavirus disease 2019 (COVID-19) is defined as illness caused by a novel coronavirus called severe acute respiratory syndrome coronavirus 2 (SARS-CoV-2; formerly called 2019-nCoV), which was first identified amid an outbreak of respiratory illness cases in Wuhan City, Hubei Province, China. It was initially reported to the WHO on December 31, 2019". In January 30, 2020, the WHO declared the COVID-19 outbreak a global health emergency. On March 11, 2020, the WHO declared COVID-19 a global pandemic, its first such designation since declaring H1N1 influenza a pandemic in 2009.

The COVID-19 pandemic caused by the severe acute respiratory syndrome coronavirus 2 (SARS-CoV-2) has caused more than six million deaths globally. (https://covid19.who.int). (Globally, as of 4:54pm CET, 23 December 2022, there have been

663,640,386 confirmed cases of COVID-19, including **6,713,093**

deaths, reported to WHO at WHO Coronavirus (COVID-19)

Dashboard). COVID-19 deaths are primarily caused by acute

respiratory distress syndrome (ARDS) and by a cytokine storm

syndrome, i.e., a state of hyper inflammation leading to multi-organ

failure [1].

One of the major challenges in fighting the pandemic has

been the lack of effective therapeutic solutions. It's not new to

anyone that for about six months after the virus was announced, the

only cure to it was prevention. Rules and precautions like use of

face masks, washing and sanitizing of hands, keeping a distance of

at least 1–2 meters (3-6 feet) apart from the next person, travel bans,

compulsory isolation for medical personnel and other professions

were only some of the rules we were subjected to. But even though

it wasn't really obvious, The World Health Organization (WHO)

had and has been working closely with global experts, governments

and partners to rapidly expand scientific knowledge on the virus, to

track the spread and virulence of the virus, and to provide advice to

countries and individuals on measures to protect health and prevent the spread of this outbreak, including authorize the medicines for COVID-19.

2.2 COVID Symptoms

People with COVID-19 have had a wide range of symptoms reported – ranging from mild symptoms to severe illness. Anyone can have mild to severe symptoms. Symptoms may appear 2-14 days after exposure to the virus. According to the Centers for Disease Control and Prevention (CDC), common COVID-19 symptoms include: Fever or chills, cough, shortness of breath or difficulty breathing, fatigue, muscle or body aches, headache, new loss of taste or smell, sore throat, congestion or runny nose, nausea or vomiting, diarrhea, e.t.c.

COVID hits everyone differently. It is the same string of virus, different people with different immune system reacted dramatically different. Someone can have COVID without any symptom-- asymptomatic. Most people infected with the virus will experience mild to moderate symptoms of headaches, fatigue, and coughing. Those people often fight the virus without any special treatment or hospitalization. Some of the short-term impacts reported by people with mild symptoms include shortness of breath, fever, cough, fatigue (tiredness), and body aches. The symptoms might last a few days. People who have the virus will most likely feel better in about a week.

For more severe cases, the virus takes on a more severe hold—that can include the development of pneumonia, a severe respiratory infection, sometimes requiring hospitalization or mechanical ventilation, and potentially even resulting in death. Short-term impacts may include respiratory (breathing) failure, confusion or other neurological problems, and kidney or heart damage due to a lack of oxygen or blood clots that can sometimes cause long-term problems. In fact, the World Health Organization (WHO) first called the virus novel coronavirus-infected pneumonia (NCIP) before shortening the name to COVID-19. The SARS-CoV-2 virus was also first identified in Wuhan, China, due to cases of "pneumonia of unknown etiology," or unknown cause, the WHO reported in January 2020.

The virus infects the airways and damages the lungs. To fight off the infection, the immune system causes inflammation, which can also cause damage and allow fluid to leak into the small air sacs of the lungs, leading to pneumonia. COVID pneumonia is a complication of COVID-19 that causes inflammation and fluid in the lungs. The symptoms of COVID-19 pneumonia are basically the same as those for other forms of pneumonia. Those include: cough, fever, shortness of breath, stabbing chest pain that gets worse when you breathe deeply or cough, loss of appetite, and fatigue. (htttps://www.health.com/condition/pneumonia/covid-19-pneumonia).

All pneumonias cause inflammation and fluid in the lungs. But research suggests that the SARS-CoV-2 virus that causes COVID pneumonia moves differently through the lungs than other viruses and bacteria that cause pneumonia. COVID pneumonia spreads across the lungs slowly, using the body's own immune system to spread, which means it tends to last longer and cause damage in more places. Other pneumonias cause acute disease — symptoms come on all at once — but don't last as long.

If COVID-19 pneumonia progresses, more of the air sacs can become filled with fluid leaking from the tiny blood vessels in the lungs. Eventually, shortness of breath sets in, and can lead to acute respiratory distress syndrome (ARDS), a form of lung failure.

Severe symptoms include hard to breath, pneumonia, failure of kidney, heart, lung, brain. According to the CDC, symptoms of COVID-19 that require emergency medical treatment include trouble breathing; persistent pain or pressure in the chest; and pale gray- or blue-colored skin, lips, or nail beds. Keep in mind, too, that this is not an exhaustive list.

National Institutes of Health (NIH) group the symptoms in the following severity of illness categories.

- *Asymptomatic or presymptomatic infection:* Individuals who test positive for SARS-CoV-2 using a virologic test (i.e., a nucleic acid amplification test [NAAT] or an antigen test) but who have no symptoms that are consistent with COVID-19.
- *Mild illness:* Individuals who have any of the various signs and symptoms of COVID-19 (e.g., fever, cough, sore throat, malaise, headache, muscle pain, nausea, vomiting, diarrhea, loss of taste and smell) but who do not have shortness of breath, dyspnea, or abnormal chest imaging.
- *Moderate illness:* Individuals who show evidence of lower respiratory disease during clinical assessment or imaging and who have an oxygen saturation measured by pulse oximetry (SpO_2) $\geq 94\%$ on room air at sea level.
- *Severe illness:* Individuals who have SpO_2 <94% on room air at sea level, a ratio of arterial partial pressure of oxygen to fraction of inspired oxygen (PaO_2/FiO_2) <300 mm Hg, a respiratory rate >30 breaths/min, or lung infiltrates >50%.
- *Critical illness:* Individuals who have respiratory

failure, septic shock, and/or multiple organ dysfunction.

2.3 SARS-CoV-2 Variants

Like other RNA viruses, SARS-CoV-2 is constantly evolving through random mutations. (https://www.covid19treatmentguidelines.nih.gov/ on 1/24/2023) New mutations can potentially increase or decrease infectiousness and virulence. In addition, mutations can increase the virus' ability to evade adaptive immune responses from past SARS-CoV-2 infection or vaccination. This viral evolution may increase the risk of reinfection or decrease the efficacy of vaccines. There is evidence that some SARS-CoV-2 variants, such as Omicron, have reduced susceptibility to plasma from people who were previously infected or immunized, as well as to certain anti-SARS-CoV-2 mAbs.

Since December 2020, the World Health Organization (WHO) has assigned Greek letter designations to several identified variants. A SARS-CoV-2 variant designated as a variant of concern (VOC) displays certain characteristics, such as increased transmissibility or virulence. In addition, vaccines and therapeutics may have decreased effectiveness against VOCs, and the mutations found in these variants may interfere with the targets of diagnostic tests. The variant of interest (VOI) designation has been used for important variants that are not fully characterized; however, organizations do not use the same variant designations, and they may define their variant designations differently. In September 2021, the CDC added a new designation for variants: variants being monitored (VBM). This refers to variants for which data indicate a potential or clear impact on approved or authorized medical countermeasures or variants associated with more severe disease or increased transmission rates. However, these variants are either no longer detected or are circulating at very low levels in the United States; therefore, they do not pose a significant and imminent risk to public health in the United States.

The Omicron variant was designated a VOC in November 2021 and rapidly became the dominant variant across the globe. The Omicron subvariants BA.1, BA.1.1, and BA.2 emerged in early to mid-2022. The subvariants BA.4 and BA.5 and, more recently, other subvariants such as BA.2.75, BA.4.6, BF.7, BQ.1, and BQ.1.1 are circulating in the United States. The newer Omicron subvariants are more transmissible than other variants and are not susceptible to some of the anti-SARS-CoV-2 mAbs that have been developed for treatment and prevention.

Earlier variants include the Alpha (B.1.1.7) variant, which was first seen in the United Kingdom and shown to be highly infectious and possibly more virulent than previously reported variants; the Beta (B.1.351) variant, which was originally identified in South Africa; the Gamma (P.1) variant, which was identified in Manaus, Brazil; and the Delta (B.1.617.2) variant, which was identified in India. Although the Alpha, Beta, Gamma, and Delta variants were previously designated as VOCs, they have largely disappeared worldwide.

2.4 Therapeutic Solution Scope.

There are mainly two approaches of COVID solutions: one is prevention and one is therapeutic treatment, the medicine to cure COVID. As one of the prevention solution, various vaccines can be written in a book alone, but they are not included in this one. This book is mainly focus on the therapeutic solution, medicine treatments for COVID.

CHAPTER 3 THERAPUTIC SOLUTON

FOR COVID

More than three years have passed since the start of the COVID-19 pandemic, which has claimed millions of lives. Unlike the early days of the pandemic, when management decisions were based on extrapolations from in vitro data, case reports and case series, clinicians are now equipped with an armamentarium of therapies based on high-quality evidence. These treatments spread across seven main therapeutic categories: anti-inflammatory agents, antivirals, antithrombotics, therapies for acute hypoxaemic respiratory failure, anti-SARS-CoV-2 (neutralizing) antibody therapies, modulators of the renin–angiotensin–aldosterone system and vitamins.

For each of these treatments, the patient population characteristics and clinical settings in which they were studied are important considerations. Although few direct comparisons have been performed, the evidence base and magnitude of benefit for anti-inflammatory and antiviral agents clearly outweigh those of other therapeutic approaches such as vitamins [44].

Two main processes are thought to drive the pathogenesis of COVID-19. Early in the clinical course, the disease is primarily driven by the replication of SARS-CoV-2. Later in the clinical course, the disease appears to be also driven by a dysregulated immune/inflammatory response to SARS-CoV-2 infection that may lead to further tissue damage and thrombosis. Based on this understanding, therapies that directly target SARS-CoV-2 are anticipated to have the greatest effect early in the course of the disease, whereas immunosuppressive, anti-inflammatory, and antithrombotic therapies are likely to be more beneficial after COVID-19 has progressed to stages characterized by hypoxemia and endothelial dysfunction. Thus, therapies for COVID-19 can be broadly categorized as targeting the virus directly including direct antivirals and antibody-based therapies in the early stage and following with targeting the host response to infection including inflammation, thrombosis, acute respiratory distress syndrome (ARDS) and renin–angiotensin–aldosterone system (RAAS) activation) next. COVID-19 related therapies include antiviral drugs, immunomodulators, neutralizing antibody therapies, cell therapies and gene therapies.

Antiviral drugs keep viruses from multiplying and are used to treat many viral infections (such as Hepatitis C, and influenza).

Neutralizing antibody therapies may help individuals fight the virus and include manufactured antibodies, animal-sourced antibody therapies, and blood-derived products such as convalescent plasma and hyperimmune globulin, which contain antibodies taken from people who have previously had COVID-19.

Immunomodulators are aimed at tamping down the body's own immune reaction to the virus, in cases where the body's reaction basically goes overboard and starts attacking the patient's own organs.

Cell therapy products include cellular immunotherapies and other types of both autologous and allogeneic cells, such as stem cells, and related products.

Gene therapy products seek to modify or manipulate the expression of a gene or to alter the biological properties of living cells for therapeutic use.

Therapies targeting SARS-CoV-2 directly include antivirals that disrupt viral replication and neutralizing antibody therapies that prevent virus entry into host cells. Antiviral medications help the body fight off harmful viruses. The drugs can ease symptoms and shorten the length of a viral infection. Neutralizing antibodies are also a potential treatment for COVID-19[6].

Oral antivirals, intravenous remdesivir, and antispike neutralizing antibodies are effective at preventing disease progression in early COVID-19. Antiviral treatment target specific parts of the virus to stop it from multiplying in the body, helping to prevent severe illness and death. There are two major ways to take antiviral drugs: by mouth or through a vein. You take oral antiviral pills at home. You get intravenous (IV) antivirals from a health care professional. Most people who become sick with COVID-19 will only have mild illness and can get better at home. The symptoms might last a few days. People who have the virus will most likely feel better in about a week. Treatment is aimed at relieving symptoms. If you test positive for COVID-19 and have mild to moderate symptoms (non-hospitalized, not requiring oxygen or an increase in home oxygen) you may be eligible for antiviral treatments including oral antivirals or an IV (intravenous or in your arm) antiviral. Explained below are some of the recommended antivirals. In recent months, several oral antiviral drugs have also been approved, which, if given early enough, appear to significantly reduce hospitalizations.

Monoclonal antibodies represent the most effective and viable therapy and/or prophylaxis option against COVID-19, and have shown a reduction of the viral load, as well as lowering hospitalizations and death rates. Monoclonal antibodies (also called moAbs or mAbs) are proteins made in laboratories that act like proteins called antibodies in our bodies. Antibodies are parts of your immune system. They seek out the antigens (foreign materials) and stick to them in order to destroy them. Laboratory-made monoclonal antibodies help stimulate your own immune system. The word "monoclonal" refers to the fact that the antibodies created in the laboratory are clones. They are exact copies of one antibody. The generic names of the products often include the letters "mab" at the end of the name.

Monoclonal antibodies have been identified as a potential therapy to prevent disease progression in patients at risk for severe disease. Most antibodies made by the human body are polyclonal, meaning that they are derived from multiple B lymphocyte lineages and have slightly different specificities for target antigens. Monoclonal antibodies, however, are produced by a single B-lymphocyte clone and are highly specific for their target antigen. Monoclonal antibodies have been in use since 1985 and have been used as therapies for malignancy, autoimmune disease, infectious organisms, and drug reversal.

Monoclonal antibodies (mAbs) that target the SARS-CoV-2 spike protein have been shown to have clinical benefits in treating SARS-CoV-2 infection. However, laboratory studies have found that the activity of anti-SARS-CoV-2 mAbs against specific variants and subvariants can vary dramatically. Because of this, these products are not expected to be effective treatments for COVID-19 in areas where the circulating variants and subvariants are resistant to mAbs.

Monoclonal antibody treatments in inpatients have been assessed and although bamlanivimab/etesevimab and casirivimab/

imdevimab combinations have improved clinical outcomes, this was only among patients without detectable antibodies to SARS-CoV-2 at randomization, and before the emergence of the Omicron variant. As the principle in the mosquito bite infection, monoclonal antibody produced from any previous variants will not work for the new variant, on the other hand, they could worsen the symptoms which have been verified from bamlanivimab and etesevimab combination. So to treat new variant such as Omicron, the antibody need to be cloned/copied from an antibody of the people who had caught Omicron and newly generated. It seemed that the FDA just simple invoked the previous antibody authorization.

Coronavirus disease 2019 (Covid-19) pneumonia is often associated with hyper inflammation. SARS-CoV-2 infection can lead to hyperinflammation characterized by abundant circulating levels of pro-inflammatory cytokines such as IL-6. Therapies targeting inflammation include immunosuppressive drugs such as glucocorticoids (for example, dexamethasone) and anti-IL-6 receptor antibodies (for example, tocilizumab).

Several antithrombotic therapies have also been trialed to address the haemostatic and thrombotic complications associated with COVID-19, whereas different methods of oxygen delivery and intubation can be employed to treat patients with ARDS.

COVID-19 can also disrupt RAAS homeostasis and drugs such as angiotensin-converting enzyme (ACE) inhibitors or angiotensin II receptor blockers are being investigated as potential therapies.

In Summary, several promising treatment options stand out as therapeutic solutions for COVID-19, including antivirals, plasma-derived drugs, monoclonal antibodies, antimalarial, cell therapy, and corticosteroids. If you test positive for COVID-19 and have mild to moderate symptoms (non-hospitalized, not requiring oxygen or an increase in home oxygen) you may be eligible for antiviral treatments including oral antivirals or an IV (intravenous or in your arm) antiviral. If you have heavy symptom and become hospitalized with severe symptoms, and need ventilator, corticosteroids may be used, such as dexamethasone, an approved corticosteroid medication, acting as an anti-inflammatory and immunosuppressant agent. In the current pandemic, dexamethasone is declared a "major development" in the fight against COVID-19. Steroidal dexamethasone was presented as the recent advancement that significantly reduces the mortality rate among severe COVID-19 cases. Corticosteroids are now recommended for patients with severe COVID-19, including those with COVID-related ARDS. Antivirals medicine such as Paxlovid and Lagevrio for mild symptom, and dexamethasone for severe symptoms are the major CDC and NIH recommended medicines to cure COVID-19. Antiviral medicine tends to be effective to treat any coronavirrus variants as long as it is a virus. Therefore, they are approved to be effective for Omicron string.

Monoclonal antibodies against SARS-CoV-2 are a clinically validated therapeutic option against COVID-19. Because rapidly emerging virus mutants are becoming the next major concern in the fight against the global pandemic, it is imperative that these therapeutic treatments provide coverage against circulating variants and do not contribute to development of treatment-induced emergent resistance.

For monoclonal antibodies that were cloned from the previous variant induced antibody won't work for the newly muted virus infection, such as omicron., same as in the mosquito bite infection theory. Early, CDC and WHO recommended many other antibody medicine such as Bamlanivimab and etesevimab, REGEN-COV etc.all are proved to be ineffective to the currently dominated Omicron string. With Omicron, for any monoclonal antibodies to work, they need to be cloned/copied from the antibody actuated by Omicron--from the antibody of person who contracted and infected by Omicorn. But it seems that the monoclonal antibldy treatment simply were halted, not continued in the proper way.

The following subsections elaborate the pron. and con. of each medicine.

3.1 PAXLOVID

WHO has made a strong recommendation Paxlovid, for mild and moderate COVID-19 patients at highest risk of hospital admission, calling it the best therapeutic choice for high-risk patients to date. PAXLOVID has been authorized for emergency use by FDA under an EUA, for the treatment of mild-to-moderate COVID-19 in adults and pediatric patients (12 years of age and older weighing at least 40 kg) with positive results of direct SARS-CoV-2 viral testing, and who are at high risk for progression to severe COVID-19, including hospitalization or death.

It is an oral antiviral pill that developed by Pfizer (https://www.paxlovid.com/). It had an 89% reduction in the risk of hospitalization and death in unvaccinated people in the clinical trial that supported the EUA, a number that was high enough to prompt the National Institutes of Health (NIH) to prioritize it over other COVID-19 treatments. Studies outside of the laboratory have since confirmed Paxlovid's effectiveness among people who have been vaccinated. It's cheaper than many other COVID-19 drugs (it's provided for free by the U.S. government while there is a public health emergency), and, perhaps most reassuring, it is expected to work against the Omicron variant.

Paxlovid is an antiviral medicine that works by stopping the virus that causes coronavirus (COVID-19) from growing and spreading in the body. It is an oral antiviral that stop the virus that causes COVID making copies of itself in the body. It consists of two separate medications packaged together. When you take your three-pill dose, two of those pills will be nirmatrelvir, which inhibits a key enzyme that the COVID virus requires in order to make functional virus particles. After nirmatrelvir treatment, the COVID virus that is released from the cells is no longer able to enter uninfected cells in the body, which, in turn, stops the infection. The other is ritonavir, a drug that was once used to treat HIV/AIDS but is now used to boost levels of antiviral medicines. As a COVID-19 treatment, ritonavir essentially shuts down nirmatrelvir's metabolism in the liver, so that it doesn't move out of your body as quickly, which means it can work longer—giving it a boost to help fight the infection. (https://www.yalemedicine.org/news/13-things-to-know-paxlovid-covid-19).

PAXLOVID consists of 2 medicines: nirmatrelvir- an oval, pink tablets and ritonavir- a white or off-white tablets. The 2 medicines are taken together 2 times each day for 5 days. It can be taken at home to help keep high-risk patients from getting so sick that they need to be hospitalized. You have to take Paxlovid within five days of developing symptoms.

You may be eligible for Paxlovid if you're aged 18 or over, you're in the highest risk group, you've had a positive lateral flow test (reported via GOV.UK or 119), you've had coronavirus (COVID-19) symptoms within the last 5 days, or 7 days if advised by a healthcare professional (https://aspr.hhs.gov/COVID-19/Therapeutics/Products/Paxlovid/Pages/default.aspx).

The highest risk group includes some people who have:

- Down's syndrome, or another chromosomal disorder that affects your immune system.

- Certain types of cancer or have received treatment for certain types of cancer.

- Sickle cell disease.

- Certain conditions affecting their blood.

- Chronic kidney disease (CKD) stage 4 or 5.

- Severe liver disease.

- Had an organ transplant.

- Certain autoimmune or inflammatory conditions (such as rheumatoid arthritis or inflammatory bowel disease).

- HIV or AIDS and have a weakened immune system.

- a condition affecting their immune system.

- a rare condition affecting the brain or nerves (multiple sclerosis, motor neurone disease, Huntington's disease or myasthenia gravis).

A doctor or specialist will confirm if you are eligible for treatment. Tell your doctor before taking this medicine if you:

- are pregnant, trying to get pregnant, or breastfeeding.

- have ever had an allergic reaction to Paxlovid, or any other medicine.

- have problems with your kidneys.

- have problems with your liver.

- are intolerant to lactose or galactose – nirmatrelvir contains a lot of lactose.

- have lactase deficiency or glucose-galactose malabsorption.

Some side effects of Pavloxid are as follows:

(https://www.paxlovid.com/side-effects):

- **Allergic Reactions.** Allergic reactions, including severe allergic reactions (known as 'anaphylaxis'), can happen in people taking PAXLOVID, even after only 1 dose. Symptoms of an allergic reaction include: hives; trouble swallowing or breathing; swelling of the mouth, lips, or face; throat tightness; hoarseness; skin rash.

- **Liver Problems.** loss of appetite, yellowing of your skin and the whites of your eyes (jaundice), dark-colored urine, pale-colored stools and itchy skin, or stomach area (abdominal) pain

- **Resistance to HIV Medicines.** If you have untreated HIV infection, PAXLOVID may lead to some HIV medicines not working as well in the future

- Other possible side effects include:
    - altered sense of taste
    - diarrhea
    - high blood pressure
    - muscle aches
    - abdominal pain
    - nausea

3.2 REMDESIVIR (VEKLURY)

WHO has updated its recommendation on remdesivir. Previously, WHO had suggested against its use in all COVID-19 patients regardless of disease severity, due to the totality of the evidence at that time showing little or no effect on mortality (https://www.ncbi.nlm.nih.gov/pmc/articles/PMC8922517/), but following publication of new data from a clinical trial looking at the outcome of admission to hospital, WHO has updated its recommendation. WHO now suggests the use of remdesivir in mild or moderate COVID-19 patients who are at high risk of

hospitalization.

In U.S., Remdesivir is the first treatment for COVID-19 to

be approved by the U.S. Food and Drug Administration (FDA). In

November 2020, the FDA issued an emergency use authorization

(EUA) for the combination of baricitinib with remdesivir, for the

treatment of suspected or laboratory confirmed COVID-19 in

hospitalized people two years of age or older requiring

supplemental oxygen, invasive mechanical ventilation, or

extracorporeal membrane oxygenation (ECMO). In January 2022,

the FDA expanded the indication for remdesivir to include its use in

non-hospitalized adults and adolescents with positive results of

direct SARS-CoV-2 viral testing, and who are not hospitalized and

have mild-to-moderate COVID-19, and are at high risk for

progression to severe COVID-19, including hospitalization or death.

In April 2022, the approval was expanded to include children 28

days of age and older weighing at least 3 kilograms (6.6 lb) with

positive results of direct SARS-CoV-2 viral testing.

(https://en.wikipedia.org/wiki/Remdesivir)

Remdesivir, sold under the brand name Veklury, is a broad-spectrum antiviral medication developed by the biopharmaceutical company Gilead Sciences. It (https://www.veklury.com/) works by stopping the virus that causes coronavirus (COVID-19) from growing and spreading in the body. It is a nucleotide prodrug of an adenosine analog. It binds to the viral RNA-dependent RNA polymerase and inhibits viral replication by terminating RNA transcription prematurely. Remdesivir has demonstrated in vitro and in vivo activity against SARS-CoV-2.1 Remdesivir retains in vitro neutralization activity against the Omicron variant and its subvariants. It's used to treat early COVID-19 infection and help to prevent more severe symptoms.

It is given through intravenous (IV) infusion one time each day for up to 10 days for hospitalized people, and 3 days for . Intravenous remdesivir is approved by the Food and Drug Administration (FDA) for the treatment of COVID-19 in adults and pediatric patients aged $\geq$28 days and weighing $\geq$3 kg. In non-hospitalized patients with mild to moderate COVID-19 who are at high risk of progressing to severe disease, remdesivir should be started within 7 days of symptom onset and administered for 3 days.

Hospitalized patients should receive remdesivir for 5 days or until hospital discharge, whichever comes first.

The treatment is recommended by the National Institute of Health to be given as soon as possible after you have tested positive for COVID-19 and within 7 days of your symptoms starting. Remdesivir can be given to most adults, and children who weigh at least 40 kg.

These common side effects of remdesivir happen in up to 1 in 10 people.

- Headache.

- Feeling sick or being sick (nausea or vomiting).

- Allergic reaction

- Increase in liver enzymes

You may be eligible for remdesivir if you're in the highest risk group below, you've had a positive lateral flow test (reported via GOV.UK or 119) or you've had coronavirus (COVID-19) symptoms within the last 7 days.

A doctor or specialist will confirm if you are eligible for treatment. Before you have this medicine, tell your doctor if you:

- are pregnant, trying to get pregnant, or breastfeeding.

- have ever had an allergic reaction to any other medicine.

- have problems with your kidneys.

- have problems with your liver.

- are immunosuppressed.

3.3 MOLNUPIRAVIR (LAGEVRIO)

Molnupiravir, also named Lagevrio, is an antiviral medication that inhibits the replication of certain RNA viruses. Molnupiravir was originally developed to treat influenza at Emory University by the university's drug innovation company, Drug Innovation Ventures at Emory (DRIVE), but was reportedly abandoned for mutagenicity concerns. It was then acquired by Miami-based company Ridgeback Biotherapeutics, which later partnered with Merck & Co. to develop the drug further. It is used to treat COVID-19 in those infected by SARS-CoV-2. It is taken by mouth.

In December 2021, the U.S. Food and Drug Administration (FDA) granted an emergency use authorization (EUA) to molnupiravir for use in certain populations where other treatments are not feasible. The emergency use authorization was only narrowly approved (13-10) because of questions about efficacy and concerns that molnupiravir's mutagenic effects could create new variants that evade immunity and prolong the COVID-19 pandemic.

Molnupiravir inhibits viral reproduction by promoting widespread mutations in the replication of viral RNA by RNA-directed RNA polymerase. The coronavirus uses RNA as its genetic material. The structure of molnupiravir resembles the nucleosides (or chemical building blocks) used to make the virus's RNA. The drug works by incorporating itself into the RNA as it's being synthesized. This results in many mutations, or changes in the RNA genetic code, introduced into the viral RNA for the virus failed to function.

Molnupiravir is an investigational medicine to treat mild-to-moderate coronavirus disease (COVID-19) in adults with positive results of direct SARS-CoV-2 viral testing who are at high risk for progression to severe COVID-19 and for whom alternative FDA-authorized COVID-19 treatments are not accessible or clinically appropriate. It is the second oral medication against COVID 19 after nirmatrelvir/ritonavir, but with a lower efficacy: about 30% (95% CI, 1–51%) against hospitalization or death in unvaccinated adults with mild or moderate COVID-19 and at least one risk factor for disease progression. It's used to treat early COVID-19 infection and help to prevent more severe symptoms.

Molnupiravir should be provided only to non-severe COVID-19 patients with the highest risk of hospitalization. These are typically people who have not received a COVID-19 vaccination, older people, people with immunodeficiency and people living with chronic diseases.

Molnupiravir is only authorized for the treatment of mild-to-moderate COVID-19 in adults 18 and older who are at high risk for progressing to severe COVID-19, including hospitalization or death. It is not authorized for children and teenagers younger than 18 years because it may affect bone and cartilage growth. Molnupiravir shouldn't be taken if you're pregnant. It can be harmful to an unborn baby and may also affect sperm, so reliable birth control is recommended if you're having sex.

This drug is also effective for the variants of COVID-19. You may be eligible for molnupiravir if you're in the highest risk group below, you're aged 18 or over, you've had a positive lateral flow test (reported via GOV.UK or 119), you've had coronavirus

(COVID-19) symptoms within the last 5 days, or 7 days if advised by a healthcare professional.

LAGEVRIO is not authorized: for use in people less than 18 years of age; for prevention of COVID-19; for patients needing hospitalization for COVID-19; for use for longer than 5 consecutive days.

Like all medicines, molnupiravir can cause side effects in some people, although not everyone gets them. The common side effects include:

- Feeling dizzy
- Headaches
- Diarrhea
- Feeling or being sick (nausea or vomiting)

3.4 DEXAMETHASONE

Dexamethasone is for severe COVID symptom and sometime, with double infections: infected with COVID and another infection. It was tested in hospitalized patients with COVID-19 in the United Kingdom's national clinical trial RECOVERY and was found to have benefits for critically ill patients. According to preliminary findings shared with WHO (and now available as a preprint), for patients on ventilators, the treatment was shown to reduce mortality by about one third, and for patients requiring only oxygen, mortality was cut by about one fifth.

Dexamethasone is a type of medicine called a steroid (corticosteroid) and is used in a wide range of conditions for its anti-inflammatory and immunosuppressant effects. Corticosteroids are a copy of a hormone your body makes naturally. "More recently, corticosteroid use in pneumonia has been associated with improved clinical outcomes, including decreased mortality in patients with SARS-CoV-2 infection and acute hypoxemic respiratory failure, specifically when given early (within 48 hours) and in a subset of patients with elevated inflammatory markers." (https://www.mayoclinic.org/medical-professionals/pulmonary-medicine/news/steroid-use-in-pneumonia/mac-20530202).

Dexamethasone is a glucocorticoid medication used to treat rheumatic problems, a number of skin diseases, severe allergies, asthma, chronic obstructive lung disease, croup, brain swelling, eye pain following eye surgery, superior vena cava syndrome, and along with antibiotics in tuberculosis. Dexamethasone may be used to treat conditions characterized by inflammation. It helps to reduce inflammation and calms down an overactive immune system. It works by mimicking the effect of cortisol, a hormone released by the adrenal glands (which are located on top of the kidneys) that controls metabolism and stress.

On 16 June, investigators on the COVID-19 recovery trial revealed in a press release that participants with severe COVID-19 (2104) given 6 mg dexamethasone once daily had an 8-26% lower mortality than 4321 participants given standard care [8].

National Institutes of Health (NIH) recommendations for the use of corticosteroids in hospitalized patients with COVID-19 who need either mechanical ventilation or supplemental oxygen (without ventilation). For people with severe COVID-19 cases, it is prescribed to take 6 mg once daily in addition to standard care for up to 10 days. Peak effects of dexamethasone are reached within 10 to 30 minutes of administration; however, it may take a couple of days before any inflammation is well controlled. "Most adults and children (including babies) can take dexamethasone".

NIH also recommended the use of the combinations of immunomodulators:

SUSAN SU © 2023

- Dexamethasone plus oral (PO) baricitinib (AI); or

- Dexamethasone plus intravenous (IV) tocilizumab (BIIa)

If PO baricitinib and IV tocilizumab are not available or not feasible to use, PO tofacitinib can be used instead of PO baricitinib (BIIa), and IV sarilumab can be used instead of IV tocilizumab (BIIa). When neither baricitinib nor tocilizumab is available or feasible to use, the JAK inhibitor tofacitinib or the IL-6 inhibitor sarilumab may be used as alternative agents for baricitinib or tocilizumab, respectively. Tofacitinib decreased the risk for respiratory failure or death in the STOP-COVID trial, and sarilumab reduced mortality and the duration of organ support to the same degree as tocilizumab in the REMAP-CAP trial. The Panel recommends using dexamethasone alone if baricitinib, tofacitinib, tocilizumab, or sarilumab cannot be obtained (AI).

National Institutes of Health (NIH) also recommended against "… the use of dexamethasone or other systemic corticosteroids to treat outpatients with mild to moderate COVID-19 who do not require hospitalization or supplemental oxygen (AIIb)". Dexamethasone is not suitable for everyone. Tell your doctor before starting on this medicine if:

- You have had an allergic reaction to dexamethasone or any other medicine in the past.

- You have recently been in contact with someone with shingles, chickenpox or measles.

- You have an infection or any unhealed wounds.

- You have liver or kidney problems.

- You have ever had mental health problems (or a close family member has).

- You have ever had tuberculosis (TB).

- You have high blood pressure, heart failure or recently had a heart attack.

- You have diabetes.

- You have epilepsy.

- You have glaucoma.

- You have an underactive thyroid.

- You have osteoporosis (thinning bones).

- You have a stomach ulcer.

- You have myasthenia gravis, a rare condition that causes muscle weakness.

- You have recently had vaccinations, or are due to have vaccinations.

- You're pregnant, trying to get pregnant or breastfeeding.

3.5 TOCILIZUMAB

Tocilizumab (TCZ), also named ACTEMRA, is an anti-IL-6R biological therapy It has been approved for the treatment of CRS and is used in patients with MAS (and in other rheumatologic conditions like Rheumatoid Arthritis (RA) or Giant Cell Arteritis (GCA). Tocilizumab (TCZ), a monoclonal antibody against interleukin-6 (IL-6), emerged as an alternative treatment for COVID-19 patients with a risk of cytokine storms recently [10]. Tocilizumab is an IV biologic medication. It works by lowering an inflammation-causing chemical in the body that can be elevated in the lungs from COVID-19. Tocilizumab is a monoclonal antibody that inhibits the Interleukin-6 (IL-6) receptor. Interleukin-6 induces an inflammatory response and is found in high levels in patients critically ill with COVID-19.

According to WHO, "Tocilizumab given intravenously has been shown in clinical studies to reduce death in certain patients with COVID-19 who are severely ill, are rapidly deteriorating and have increasing oxygen needs, and who have a significant inflammatory response. In the largest clinical trial recovery, tocilizumab also reduced patients' time in hospital.".

Tocilizumab may ameliorate the inflammatory manifestations associated with severe coronavirus disease 2019 (COVID-19) and thus improve clinical outcomes. Tocilizumab is an effective treatment in severe patients of COVID-19 to calm the inflammatory storm and reduce mortality [13]. It is most effective when used within 10 days of developing symptoms.

WHO recommends tocilizumab only for patients diagnosed with severe or critical COVID-19. It should be administered by a healthcare worker in a monitored clinical setting along with the current standard of care for COVID-19, which includes oxygen, corticosteroids, and other medications. ACTEMRA is FDA approved for the treatment of adults hospitalized with COVID-19 who are receiving systemic corticosteroids and require supplemental oxygen, non-invasive or invasive mechanical ventilation, or extracorporeal membrane oxygenation (ECMO). FDA has issued an Emergency Use Authorization (EUA) for use of ACTEMRA to treat coronavirus disease 2019 (COVID-19) in pediatric patients (two years of age and older) who are in the hospital and who are receiving corticosteroids and require supplemental oxygen, or a machine that helps with their breathing (ventilator) or a machine that adds oxygen to the blood outside the body (extracorporeal membrane oxygenation or ECMO).

ACTEMRA changes the way your immune system works. This can make you more likely to get infections or make any current infection worse. Some people have serious infections while taking ACTEMRA, including tuberculosis (TB), and infections caused by bacteria, fungi, or viruses that can spread throughout the body. Some people have died from these infections. Before starting ACTEMRA, tell your healthcare provider if you have:

- an infection, think you may have an infection, are being treated for an infection, or get a lot of infections that return. Symptoms of an infection, with or without a fever, include sweating or chills; shortness of breath; warm, red or painful skin or sores on your body; feeling very tired; muscle aches; blood in phlegm; diarrhea or stomach pain;

cough; weight loss; burning when you urinate or urinating more than normal

- any of the following conditions that may give you a higher chance of getting infections: diabetes, HIV, or a weak immune system

- tuberculosis (TB), or have been in close contact with someone with TB

- live or have lived, or have traveled to certain parts of the United States where there is an increased chance of getting fungal infections. These parts include the Ohio and Mississippi River valleys and the Southwest

- hepatitis B or have had hepatitis B

The most common side effects are:

- a cough or sore throat, blocked or runny nose.

- headaches or dizziness.

- mouth ulcers.

- high blood pressure.

- Hypercholesterolemia (increased cholesterol in the blood).

- allergic reactions - this can include aching muscles, feeling out of breath, having a tight chest, wheezing, and a high temperature.

- weight gain or swollen ankles.

- skin rashes, infections or itching.

- stomach irritation or abdominal pain.

3.6 ANAKINRA

Anakinra is a immunosuppressive drug for hyperinflammatory conditions and has been shown to be highly effective in the treatment of cytokine storm syndromes, including macrophage activation syndrome and cytokine release syndrome [14]. It has been used to treat rheumatoid arthritis and patients with severe viral infection (EBV, H1N1 and Ebola) [15]. It is through an under-the-skin (subcutaneous) injection. This medication helps manage lung inflammation by blocking a similar chemical to tocilizumab. Called IL-1, this chemical is thought to be part of an overactive immune response in COVID-19. In a study called SAVE-MORE, people receiving anakinra were less likely to develop severe COVID-19 after 28 days.

Anakinra is prescribed for hospitalized adults who require supplemental oxygen, a ventilator, or who need extracorporeal membrane oxygenation (ECMO; a device that adds oxygen to the blood).

Anakinra is authorized to treat hospitalized adults with pneumonia caused by COVID-19. But it should only be given to adults who need supplemental oxygen, are at risk for severe respiratory failure, and likely have a high amount of a specific inflammatory protein.

Coronaviruses can induce the production of interleukin (IL)-1β, IL-6, tumour necrosis factor, and other cytokines implicated in autoinflammatory disorders. It has been postulated that anakinra, a recombinant IL-1 receptor antagonist, might help to neutralize the severe acute respiratory syndrome coronavirus 2 (SARS-CoV-2) related hyperinflammatory state, which is considered to be one cause of acute respiratory distress among patients with COVID-19[17].

Some of the side effects that were noticed are: redness, swelling, bruising, itching, or pain at the site of injection; headache, nausea, vomiting, diarrhea, runny nose, stomach pain, joint pain.

Some side effects can be serious. If you experience any of these symptoms or those listed in the section, call your doctor immediately or get emergency medical treatment: rash, itching, hives, swelling of the lips, tongue, mouth, or face, dizziness, fainting, difficulty breathing, wheezing, sweating, fast or racing heart beat.

3.7 BARICITINIB

Baricitinib (Olumiant™) is an orally-administered, small-molecule, janus-associated kinase (JAK) inhibitor developed by Eli Lilly and Incyte Corporation for the treatment of rheumatoid arthritis (RA), atopic dermatitis and systemic lupus erythematosus. It's classified as a Janus kinase (JAK) inhibitor, and it works by lowering inflammation in the body.

In November 2020, the FDA issued an emergency use authorization (EUA) for the combination of baricitinib with remdesivir, for the treatment of suspected or laboratory confirmed COVID-19 in hospitalized people aged two years of age or older requiring supplemental oxygen, invasive mechanical ventilation, or extracorporeal membrane oxygenation (ECMO). In May 2022, the

FDA approved baricitinib for the treatment of COVID-19 in hospitalized adults requiring supplemental oxygen, non-invasive or invasive mechanical ventilation, or extracorporeal membrane oxygenation (ECMO). Baricitinib is the first immunomodulatory treatment for COVID-19 to receive FDA approval. In the United States, baricitinib is authorized under an emergency use authorization (EUA) for the treatment of COVID-19 in hospitalized people aged 2 to less than 18 years of age who require supplemental oxygen, non-invasive or invasive mechanical ventilation, or extracorporeal membrane oxygenation. As of January 2022, the World Health Organization strongly recommended baricitinib for patients with severe or critical COVID-19.

A hyperinflammatory response to severe acute respiratory syndrome - coronavirus 2 (SARS-CoV-2) infection, reminiscent of cytokine release syndrome, has been implicated in the pathophysiology of acute respiratory distress syndrome and organ damage in patients with coronavirus disease 2019 (COVID-19). Agents that inhibit components of the proinflammatory cascade have garnered interest as potential treatment options, with hopes that dampening the proinflammatory process may improve clinical outcomes.

Baricitinib is a reversible Janus - associated kinase (JAK)-inhibitor that interrupts the signaling of multiple cytokines implicated in COVID-19 immunopathology. It may also have antiviral effects by targeting host factors that viruses rely on for cell entry and by suppressing type I interferon driven angiotensin-converting-enzyme-2 up regulation.

However, baricitinib carries the risk of increased thromboembolic events, which is concerning given the proclivity towards a hypercoagulable state in patients with COVID-19[18]. Baricitinib is only meant to treat certain people with severe COVID-19 who are in the hospital.

Clinical trials (ACTT-2 and COV-BARRIER) and real world studies both show that baricitinib can help lower the risk of death due to COVID-19 when used alongside other treatments in the hospital.

Along with its needed effects, baricitinib may cause some unwanted effects. Upper respiratory tract infections and high blood cholesterol levels (hypercholesterolemia) occurred in more than

10% of patients. Less common side effects included other infections such as herpes zoster, herpes simplex, urinary tract infections, and gastroenteritis. Although not all of these side effects may occur, if they do occur, they may need medical attention. Check with your doctor immediately if any of the following side effects occur: Body aches or pain, chest tightness, chills, cough, difficulty in breathing, ear congestion, fever, headache, hoarseness, loss of voice, muscle aches, pain or tenderness around the eyes and cheekbones, runny or stuffy nose, sneezing, sore throat, trouble in swallowing, unusual tiredness or weakness, black, tarry stools, bladder pain, blemishes on the skin, bloody or cloudy urine, burning, itching, and pain in hairy areas, pus at the root of the hair, chest pain or tightness, cough producing mucus, difficult, burning, or painful urination, frequent urge to urinate, itching of the vagina or outside genitals, lower back or side pain, pain, redness, or swelling in the arm or leg, pain during sexual intercourse, pains in the chest, groin, or legs, especially calves of the legs, pale skin, pimples, severe headaches of sudden onset, stomach pain, sudden loss of coordination, sudden onset of slurred speech, sudden vision changes, thick, white curd-like vaginal discharge without odor or with mild odor, trouble breathing, unusual bleeding or bruising, anxiety, burning or stinging of the skin, coughing or spitting up blood, dizziness or lightheadedness, increased weight, night sweats, painful blisters on the trunk of the body, painful cold sores or blisters on the lips, nose, eyes, or genitals, sudden high fever or low-grade fever for months, chest discomfort, confusion, difficulty in speaking, double vision, inability to move the arms, legs, or facial muscles, inability to speak, large, hive-like swelling on the face, eyelids, lips, tongue, throat, hands, legs, feet, or sex organs; nausea; no blood pressure or pulse; pain or discomfort in the arms, jaw, back or neck; persistent non-healing sore; pink growth; reddish patch or irritated area; shiny bump; stopping of heart; sweating; unconsciousness; white, yellow, or waxy scar-like area.

3.8 BAMLANIVIMAB/ETESEVIMAB

Bamlanivimab/etesevimab is a combination of two monoclonal antibodies, bamlanivimab and etesevimab, administered together via intravenous infusion as a treatment for COVID-19. Eli Lilly licensed etesevimab from Junshi Biosciences. However, in Lilly's website, it says "Due to high frequency of the Omicron variant, bamlanivimab and etesevimab are not currently authorized in any U.S. region". (https://www.covid19.lilly.com/bam-ete).

Bamlanivimab and etesevimab together have not been approved, but have been authorized for emergency use by the FDA. In February 2021, the FDA issued an emergency use authorization (EUA) for bamlanivimab and etesevimab administered together for the treatment of mild to moderate COVID-19 in people twelve years of age or older weighing at least 40 kilograms (88 lb) who test positive for SARS-CoV-2 and who are at high risk for progressing to severe COVID-19. The authorized use includes treatment for those who are 65 years of age or older or who have certain chronic medical conditions. While bamlanivimab and etesevimab administered together resulted in a lower risk of resistant viruses developing during treatment compared with bamlanivimab administered alone, both treatments are available under an EUA and are expected to benefit people at high risk of disease progression. On 16 April 2021, the FDA revoked the emergency use authorization (EUA) that allowed for the investigational monoclonal antibody therapy bamlanivimab, when administered alone, to be used for the treatment of mild-to-moderate COVID-19 in adults and certain pediatric patients. In January 2022, the U.S. Food and Drug Administration (FDA) revised the authorizations for two monoclonal antibody treatments – bamlanivimab/etesevimab (administered together) and casirivimab/imdevimab – to limit their use to only when the recipients are likely to have been infected with or exposed to a variant that is susceptible to these treatments.[11] Because data show these treatments are highly unlikely to be active against the omicron variant.

Neutralizing monoclonal antibodies (mAbs), as bamlanivimab and etesevimab, have been shown to benefit certain subpopulations after exposure to severe acute respiratory syndrome coronavirus 2 (SARS-CoV-2). They work by binding to different parts of the virus' spike protein, preventing it from entering and infecting your cells. Unlike vaccine-derived immunity that develops over time, administration of neutralizing mAbs is an immediate and passive immunotherapy, with the potential to reduce disease progression, emergency room visits, hospitalizations, and death. Bamlanivimab alone and together with etesevimab hold emergency use authorizations in several countries globally, with countries increasingly transitioning to the use of bamlanivimab and etesevimab together and other authorized mAbs on the basis of their evolving variant landscape, regulatory authorizations, and access to drugs. However, bamlanivimab and etesevimab aren't recommended due to resistance concerns with the Omicron variant.

Both medications are infused into the vein at the same time as a single infusion. Bamlanivimab and etesevimab, administered together, may only be used as post-exposure prophylaxis for adults and pediatric patients (12 years of age and older weighing at least 40 kg) who are:

- at high risk for progression to severe COVID-19, including hospitalization or death, and

- not fully vaccinated or who are not expected to mount an adequate immune response to complete SARS-CoV-2 vaccination (for example, people with immunocompromising conditions, including those taking immunosuppressive medications), and have been exposed to an individual infected with SARS-CoV-2 consistent with close contact criteria per Centers for Disease Control and Prevention.

- Or, who are at high risk of exposure to an individual infected with SARS-CoV-2 because of occurrence of SARS-

CoV-2 infection in other individuals in the same institutional setting (for example, nursing homes or prisons)

Serious hypersensitivity reactions, including anaphylaxis, have been observed with administration of bamlanivimab and etesevimab. Infusion reactions during and within 24 hours after the infusion. Sometimes, these may be severe or life-threatening.

As the principle in mosquito bite, if one is infected by a different or a newly mutated string of coronavirus, injecting the antibody from a previous one could worsen the symptom. Worsening of COVID-19 has happened after the use of drugs like this one. Symptoms included fever, trouble breathing, fast or slow heartbeat, or feeling confused, tired, or weak. It is not known if this was related to the use of these drugs.

Either before taking this medication or when you're taking this medication, tell your healthcare providers during every appointment. These are some side effects that may occur after using this drug:

- Signs of an allergic reaction, like rash; hives; itching; red, swollen, blistered, or peeling skin with or without fever; wheezing; tightness in the chest or throat; trouble breathing, swallowing, or talking; unusual hoarseness; or swelling of the mouth, face, lips, tongue, or throat.

- Fever or chills; chest pain or pressure; fast, slow, or abnormal heartbeat; upset stomach; shortness of breath or wheezing; signs of high or low blood pressure like headache, dizziness, or passing out; throat irritation; muscle aches; swelling of your lips, face, or throat; sweating a lot; or any other bad effects during or within 24 hours after the infusion.

3.9 REGEN-COV

REGEN-COV website (regencov.com") says that "On January 24, 2022, the U.S. Food and Drug Administration (FDA) amended the Emergency Use Authorization (EUA) for REGEN-COV to exclude its use in geographic regions where, based on available information including variant susceptibility and regional variant frequency, infection or exposure is likely due to a variant such as Omicron (B.1.1.529) that is not susceptible to the treatment. With this EUA revision, REGEN-COV is not currently authorized for use in any U.S. states, territories or jurisdictions, since Omicron is currently the dominant variant across the United States. REGEN-COV remains an investigational drug and is not approved for any indication".

REGEN-CON, also known as "Ronapreve," is a combination of two monoclonal antibodies casirivimab and imdevimab. The combination of two antibodies is intended to prevent mutational escape. It was developed by the American biotechnology company Regeneron Pharmaceuticals. Similar to Bamlanivimab/etesevimab monoclonal antibodies combination, it only treated early COVID strings, preventing it from entering and infecting the cells. They do not work for the newly muted strings such as Omicron. In January 2022, the U.S. Food and Drug Administration (FDA) revised the authorizations for two monoclonal antibody treatments – bamlanivimab/etesevimab (administered together) and casirivimab/imdevimab – to limit their use to only when the recipients are likely to have been infected with or exposed to a variant that is susceptible to these treatments because data show these treatments are highly unlikely to be active against the omicron variant.

REGEN-CON is an IV treatment that includes two monoclonal antibody medications: casirivimab and imdevimab. The combination works by targeting the SARS-CoV-2 spike protein, inhibiting its interaction with the human angiotensin-converting enzyme 2 (ACE2) receptors, and eliminating the virus. Early clinical trial showed that REGEN-COV reduced the viral load and number of medical visits in patients with early coronavirus infection. It has been shown to markedly reduce the risk of hospitalization or death among high-risk persons with coronavirus disease 2019.

REGEN-COV acquired its first emergency use license in the United States to treat COVID-19 on November 21st, 2020. On 21 November 2020, the U.S. Food and Drug Administration (FDA) issued an emergency use authorization (EUA) for casirivimab and imdevimab to be administered together for the treatment of mild to moderate [COVID-19] in people twelve years of age or older weighing at least 40 kilograms (88 lb) with positive results of direct SARS-CoV-2 viral testing and who are at high risk for progressing to severe COVID-19.[9][23][12][36] This includes those who are 65 years of age or older or who have certain chronic medical conditions.[9] Casirivimab and imdevimab must be administered together by intravenous (IV) infusion or subcutaneous injection. n July 2021, the U.S. FDA revised the emergency use authorization (EUA) for REGEN-COV (casirivimab and imdevimab, administered together) authorizing REGEN-COV for emergency use as post-exposure prophylaxis (prevention) for COVID-19 in people aged twelve years of age and older weighing at least 40 kilograms (88 lb) who are at high risk for progression to severe COVID-19, including hospitalization or death. REGEN-COV remains authorized for the treatment of mild-to-moderate COVID-19 in people aged twelve years of age and older weighing at least 40 kilograms (88 lb) with positive results of direct SARS-CoV-2 viral testing, and who are at high risk for progression to severe COVID-19, including hospitalization or death.

In a separate study, the combination of casirivimab and imdevimab reduced hospital admission or mortality in high-risk non-admitted patients by 70% in a phase III trial. For the novel Omicron type of SARS-CoV-2, a combination of monoclonal antibodies has been reported as ineffective.

The main adverse effects reported for REGEN-COV were dizziness, nausea, rash, chills, and lymphadenopathy. Whereas flushing, urticaria, anaphylaxis, and pruritus were rarely reported.

Previously, REGEN-COV can be infused into the vein outside the hospital and it can also be injected under the skin. REGEN-COV has been approved as a treatment for high-risk patients infected with SARS-CoV-2 within five days of their diagnosis.

Hospitalized patients with Covid-19 experience high mortality rates, ranging from 10-30%. Casirivimab and imdevimab (REGEN-COV®) is authorized in various jurisdictions for use in outpatients with Covid-19 and in post-exposure prophylaxis. The UK-based platform RECOVERY study reported improved survival in hospitalized seronegative patients treated with REGEN-COV, but in most of the world, anti-spike monoclonal antibody therapy is currently not approved for use in hospitalized patients [25]. Some warnings and precautions are: hypersensitivity Including anaphylaxis and infusion-Related Reactions: Serious hypersensitivity reactions, including anaphylaxis, have been observed with administration of REGEN-COV. Hypersensitivity reactions occurring more than 24 hours after the infusion have also been reported with the use of REGEN-COV under EUA. Infusion-related reactions, occurring during the infusion and up to 24 hours after the infusion, have been observed with administration of REGEN-COV. These reactions may be severe or life-threatening. Signs and symptoms of infusion-related reactions may include: fever, difficulty breathing, reduced oxygen saturation, chills, nausea, arrhythmia (e.g., atrial fibrillation, tachycardia, bradycardia), chest pain or discomfort, weakness, altered mental status, headache, bronchospasm, hypotension, hypertension, angioedema, throat irritation, rash including urticaria, pruritus, myalgia, vasovagal reactions (e.g., pre-syncope, syncope), dizziness, fatigue and diaphoresis.

Clinical worsening of COVID-19 after administration of REGEN-COV has been reported and may include signs or symptoms of fever, hypoxia or increased respiratory difficulty, arrhythmia (e.g., atrial fibrillation, tachycardia, bradycardia), fatigue, and altered mental status. Some of these events requires hospitalization.

Monoclonal antibodies, such as REGEN-COV, may be associated with worse clinical outcomes when administered to hospitalized patients with COVID-19 requiring high-flow oxygen or mechanical ventilation. Therefore, REGEN-COV is not authorized for use in patients who are hospitalized due to COVID-19, OR who require oxygen therapy due to COVID-19, OR who require an increase in baseline oxygen flow rate due to COVID-19 in those on chronic oxygen therapy due to underlying non-COVID-19–related comorbidity.

REGEN-COV was previously available to treat mild-to-moderate COVID-19 and for PEP in people ages 12 and older who were at high risk of severe illness. REGEN-COV isn't currently recommended due to resistance concerns with the Omicron variant.

3.10 SARILUMAB

Sarilumab, sold under the brand name Kevzara, is a human monoclonal antibody medication against the interleukin-6 receptor. Regeneron Pharmaceuticals and Sanofi developed the drug for the treatment of rheumatoid arthritis (RA). Sarilumab is a type of drug called a biological therapy. Sarilumab, initially approved for use in rheumatoid arthritis. Additionally, this drug has been considered for off-label use in the treatment of COVID-19. Tocilizumab seems to be more beneficial, whereas the clinical efficacy of Sarilumab has not been established as data on decreased mortality was often not significant. The number of trials did not allow for the identification of a specific patient subset that benefits the most from Sarilumab treatment, yet (May 2022).

Sarilumab comes as an injection under the skin, known as a subcutaneous injection, once every two weeks. This is done using either a pre-filled syringe or an injector pen.

The most common side effects aren't usually serious – they include:

- a cough or sore throat.

- a blocked or runny nose.

- cold sores.

- urinary tract infections.

- redness and itching at the site of the injection.

Sarilumab can make you more likely to pick up infections and it can also make them harder to spot. Tell your doctor or rheumatology nurse if you develop a sore throat or fever, or have unexplained bruising, bleeding or paleness. You should also tell them if you have any other new symptoms.

3.11 SOTROVIMAB

Sotrovimab, sold under the brand name Xevudy, is a human neutralizing monoclonal antibody with activity against severe acute COVID-19. It was developed by GlaxoSmithKline and Vir Biotechnology, Inc. Sotrovimab is designed to attach to the spike protein of SARS-CoV-2. Although Sotrovimab was used world-wide against SARS-CoV-2, including in the United States under an FDA emergency use authorization (EUA), the FDA canceled the EUA in April 2022 due to lack of efficacy against the Omicron variant.

Sotrovimab is given by intravenous infusion, preferably within 5 days of onset of COVID-19 symptoms.

3.12 CONVALESCENT PLASMA

Convalescent plasma therapy uses blood from people who've recovered from an illness to help others recover. Plasma from donors who have recovered from COVID-19 contain antibodies to SARS-CoV-2 that could help suppress viral replication. Blood donated by people who've recovered from

COVID-19 has antibodies to the virus that causes it. The donated blood is processed to remove blood cells, leaving behind liquid (plasma) and antibodies. These can be given to people with COVID-19 to boost their ability to fight the virus.

In August 2020, the Food and Drug Administration (FDA) issued an Emergency Use Authorization (EUA) for COVID-19 convalescent plasma (CCP) for the treatment of hospitalized patients with COVID-19. The EUA was subsequently revised on December 27, 202. The current EUA limits the authorization to the use of CCP products that contain high levels of anti-SARS-CoV-2 antibodies (i.e., high-titer products) for the treatment of outpatients or inpatients with COVID-19 who have immunosuppressive disease or who are receiving immunosuppressive treatment.

WHO has updated its living guideline on COVID-19 therapeutics to include convalescent plasma. For non-severe COVID-19 patients, WHO recommends against its use, while it should only be used within clinical trials for severe and critical COVID-19 patients. Current evidence shows that convalescent plasma does not improve survival or reduce the need for mechanical ventilation, while it has significant costs. While the evidence that convalescent plasma has no benefit in non-severe patients was certain, it was less so in the case of severe and critically ill patients. Also antibody may help to attack the virus, but not the inflammation.

Blood has been used to treat many other conditions. It's usually very safe. The risk of getting COVID-19 from convalescent plasma hasn't been tested yet. But researchers believe that the risk is low because donors have fully recovered from the infection. The available data suggest that serious adverse reactions following the administration of CCP are infrequent and consistent with the risks associated with plasma infusions for other indications. These risks include transfusion-transmitted infections (e.g., HIV, hepatitis B, hepatitis C), allergic reactions, anaphylactic reactions, febrile nonhemolytic reactions, transfusion-related acute lung injury, transfusion-associated circulatory overload, and hemolytic reactions. Hypothermia, metabolic complications, and post-transfusion purpura have also been described. Additional risks of CCP transfusion include a theoretical risk of antibody-dependent enhancement of SARS-CoV-2 infection.

The evolution of mutant strains such as Omicron, resistant to the most widely available anti-spike monoclonal antibodies (see above), and the lack of availability of monoclonal antibodies in many countries worldwide have the potential to rekindle use of CCP.

3.13 SABIZABULIN

Some of the antibody drugs are not effective against the omicron variant. Paxlovid is for treating mild COVID symptoms. An effective and safe oral therapeutic medicine can effectively prevent deaths in hospitalized patients with moderate to severe COVID-19 symptoms is desperately needed. Sabizabulin with its anti-viral and anti-inflammatory properties might be the solution- an oral therapy for hospitalized COVID-19 patients with serious illness.

Severe COVID-19 is thought to be driven by excess inflammation. Sabizabulin is a novel microtubule disruptor that has dual antiviral and anti-inflammatory activities in preclinical models. Like colchicine, it binds to microtubules and disrupts polymerization.

Sabizabulin is being evaluated for the treatment of cancer and, because of its antiviral and anti-inflammatory effects, now COVID-19. In June 2022, Veru sought emergency use authorization (EUA) from the US Food and Drug Administration (FDA) for the therapy. Veru Inc. recently announced the US FDA has granted Fast Track designation to the Phase 3 registration program for the investigation of sabizabulin, a novel, proprietary, oral cytoskeleton disruptor with both anti-viral and anti-inflammatory properties, to combat COVID-19 infection and the cytokine storm that is responsible for Acute Respiratory Distress Syndrome (ARDS) and death. However, on 11/9/2022, A panel of outside advisers to the U.S. health regulator voted against authorizing Sabizabulin for treating high-risk patients hospitalized with COVID-19, citing multiple concerns over efficacy and safety data being based on a small trial. The panel voted 8-5 against the oral drug sabizabulin's usage and hinted that Veru gather additional data, preferably from a larger sample, regarding the drug's ability to treat COVID-19.

As today, Sabizabulin is still pending FDA Emergency Use Authorization for treatment of hospitalized patients with COVID-19 at high risk for acute respiratory distress syndrome (ARDS)

CHAPTER 4 HOME TREATMENT FOR COVID

If you develop mild symptoms of coronavirus disease 2019 (COVID-19) or you've been exposed to the COVID-19 virus, your health care provider will recommend that you recover at home- stay in home isolation for a period of time. In the U.S., anyone who is tested positive for COVID, is advised to stay at home and self-quarantined. So if one person in the house is tested positive, then the challenge is how to prevent the virus from infecting the entire household. This Chapter provide several simple, yet effective home COVID prevention and treatment solutions.

4.1 EFFECTIVE HOME COVID PREVENTION AND TREATMENT

Open Onion

While the prevention for COVID is widely advocated as wearing the mask, keeping physical distance and vaccine, a story during the Spanish Flu gave us insight for a simple solution for COVID home prevention.

Here goes the story: The 1918 "Spanish Flu" pandemic, claimed million people death and infected multiple million people globally while no one from one household had ever caught the virus. The reason is that the house wife hanged a cut-opened onion at the door. An opened onion absorbs all kind of virus in the air-- that include the "Spanish Flu" virus, and now coronavirus.

Putting an open onion at your desk, light stand, counter will keep you from ever getting sick of any flu or coronavirus. Especially, if someone in your house is test positive and stay at home, even he/she stays in only one room, the air conditioner could take the virus in that room to circulate in the entire house. So open onion everywhere is very effective to absorb the coronavirus and keep everyone else from catching it.

Salt Lemon Water

So you fail to keep the virus off from the air; in fact, the viruses are everywhere in the air; and now you catch one too. You can quickly do something to kill the virus at your nose or throat before the it gets into your body and start to multiply itself--making babies virus) and your body's white cells have to fight and clear them.

If you feel that you catch the coronavirus, to drink salt and lemon water will kill the virus in the breather tube before it resides in your body, and your immune system have to fight to kill it which cause the inflammation.

Salt water is also a perfect way for prevent catching coronavirus. If one keeps clear the throat and month with salt water daily, there will be no chance for the virus to go anywhere to survive even if one catches it.

Vitamin C & D, Ginger + Brown Sugar

Now, even more common, you fail to clear the virus in the air, also fail to get rid of them as they enter your nose, and throat. You caught a coronavirus and that virus now comfortably resides in your body, and starts to make lots of baby virus --multiplies itself. Soon, they are all in your blood, circulating the entire body. You are infected. So, now it is your body's own immune system's become active and start to produce a lot of white cells who will fight and kill the virus cell, try to clear them. You experience a high fever and some or all of these described symptoms.

You want to do something now to make your immune system, your body fighter stronger-- to boost your immune system.

Vitamin C and D can boost your immune system. do that. Besides that, one food is a super booster, called Ginger, yes ginger. The simple effective way is to boil slice of ginger with brown sugar for thirty minutes and drink the ginger tea, it will boost your immune system dramatically.

BanLanGen

Now your body's immune system is fighting with the virus, you get a fever, also a cough--or more symptoms. Counter medicine for cold can help, such as Banlangen which has antipyretic and anti-inflammatory effects. BanLanGen can not only eliminate the toxins produced by the metabolism of bacteria in the body, thereby avoiding symptoms such as fever, but also significantly reduce the adverse reactions caused by the use of antibiotics.

4.2 HOME CARE FOR COVID

At home, you can do the following to stop the virus from infecting your body at the beginning stage.

- Rest: Your body needs rest to recover from the stress of a COVID-19 infection. The disease stresses many of your vital physical systems, including your lungs, heart, and kidneys. You can take some of the load off by conserving energy and resting up.

- Fluids: Drinking water and clear liquid beverages are important even if you do not feel thirsty. drink enough so your pee is light yellow and clear. You need to replace your body's fluid losses and thin your respiratory secretions. When you are dehydrated, your respiratory secretions thicken and are hard to clear from your lungs. Being unable to clear your secretions from your lungs may lead to pneumonia.

- Pain relievers: Taking pain relievers, such as paracetamol or ibuprofen can help relieve the symptoms of viruses. They also block the release of certain chemicals, resulting in a change in how the body reacts to pain.

At home, you can also do the following things to less the symptoms.

Treating a cough

- Avoid lying on your back. Lie on your side or sit upright.
- Try having a teaspoon of honey plus lemon. But do not give honey to babies under 12 months.

- Contact a pharmacist for advice about cough treatments.

Things to try if you're feeling breathless

If you're feeling breathless, it can help to keep your room cool. Try turning the heating down or opening a window. Do not use a fan as it may spread the virus. You could also try:

- Breathing slowly in through your nose and out through your mouth, with your lips together, like you're gently blowing out a candle.

- Sitting upright in a chair.

- Relaxing your shoulders, so you're not hunched.

- Leaning forward slightly – support yourself by putting your hands on your knees or on something stable like a chair.

Most importantly, try not to panic if you're feeling breathless. This can make it worse.

4.3 Food Fighting COVID

Besides Ginger, there are more foods that are advised to eat when fighting COVID-19 symptoms.

Avocados:

Avocados are rich in glutathione. Glutathione helps reduce oxidative stress by either stimulating or reducing the body's immunological response. Inflammation can be a culprit of symptoms like muscle aches, fever, fatigue, and a sore throat. In addition to low glutathione, low potassium is commonly found in people with the COVID-19 infection, and symptoms can include constipation, fatigue, muscle weakness or spasms, and heart palpitations. Avocados are also high in potassium with 21% of your daily value in just one fruit. This can help replenish your potassium stores.

Yogurt

Yogurt, kefir, and other probiotic foods can help restore the healthy bacteria in your gut, helping you feel better and reducing the chances of subsequent infections and illness while you're recovering from COVID-19 or after. COVID-19 drastically alters the gut microbiome. So during and after COVID-19, a quality probiotic is essential.

Jalapeño peppers

If you have a persistent cough, eating spicy peppers like jalapeños that are rich in capsaicin could help. A small January

2015 study in Respiratory Medicine found that chronic coughs decreased in people who took capsaicin powder daily for four weeks. But, if you also have a runny nose, keep in mind that spicy foods could worsen this symptom, as it loosens mucus.

Watermelon:

If you're having trouble drinking enough fluids, try eating foods high in water and other important nutrients. Watermelon is over 90% water, and a good source of vitamin A and vitamin C. Additionally, it has 11 grams of carbohydrates to help you feel more energized. Staying hydrated will help thin mucous, relieve sore muscles, and help improve headaches.

Chicken soup:

Chicken noodle soup is the classic sick day food, and there's actually a scientific reason why. In 2000, researchers at the University of Nebraska Medical Center put chicken soup to the test and found a mild anti-inflammatory effect from the chicken soup that actually helped inhibit neutrophil products, which are a known cause of mucous production in respiratory infections like COVID.

Tuna fish:

If you're feeling up to it, tuna fish can be key to feeling better and fighting off the symptoms of COVID-19. Tuna, especially albacore tuna, is high in omega-3 fatty acids and vitamin C, which can help lower inflammation in the body. An April 2022 article in the International Journal of General Medicine reports that in severe cases of COVID-19, omega-3 fatty acid supplementation could be useful in reducing the duration of symptoms, most likely related to their inflammation-reducing effects. Also, an October 2022 study in Life Sciences found that people treated with vitamin D had lower levels of inflammatory markers in their blood, which also led to shorter ICU stays. Canned tuna is easy to get and prepare as well if you're not feeling well enough to cook. Mix a can of tuna fish with avocado and enjoy it on a whole wheat pita for an easy and nutrient-rich lunch.

CHAPTER 5 POST-COVID CARE AND

TREATMENT

5.1 POST-COVID CONDITION

Post COVID-19 condition, also known as "long COVID," refers collectively to the constellation of long-term symptoms that some people experience after they have had COVID-19. People who experience post COVID-19 condition sometimes refer to themselves as "long-haulers.". WHO defined it as "Post COVID-19 condition is defined as the illness that occurs in people who have a history of probable or confirmed SARS-CoV-2 infection; usually within three months from the onset of COVID-19, with symptoms and effects that last for at least two months. The symptoms and effects of post COVID-19 condition cannot be explained by an alternative diagnosis.

People call post-COVID conditions by many names, including: Long COVID, long-haul COVID, post-acute COVID-19, post-acute sequelae of SARS CoV-2 infection (PASC), long-term effects of COVID, and chronic COVID.

While most people get over with COVID, completely recovered in week, many people caught COVID suffer long term side effect. Some people develop a variety of mid- and long-term effects like fatigue, breathlessness and cognitive dysfunction (for example, confusion, forgetfulness, or a lack of mental focus and clarity). Some people also experience psychological effects as part of post COVID-19 condition. These symptoms might persist from their initial illness or develop after their recovery. They can come and go or relapse over time. WHO estimated that "approximately 10%-20% of people experience a variety of mid- and long-term effects after they recover from their initial illness.

Most people with COVID-19 get better within a few days to a few weeks after infection, so at least four weeks after infection is the start of when post-COVID conditions could first be identified. Most people with post-COVID conditions experienced symptoms days after first learning they had COVID-19, but some people who later experienced post-COVID conditions may not have tested positive for the virus or did not know when they got infected. Even a patient who recovers from an asymptomatic or mild case of COVID-19 is at risk of developing one or more Post-COVID Conditions.

People with post-COVID conditions can have a wide range of symptoms that can last weeks, months, or even years after infection. Although most patients' symptoms slowly improve with time. People with post COVID-19 condition may have difficulty functioning in everyday life. Their condition may affect their ability to perform daily activities such as work or household chores, and sometimes result in disability.

Post-COVID conditions may not affect everyone the same way. People with post-COVID conditions may experience health problems from different types and combinations of symptoms happening over different lengths of time.

Post-COVID conditions are found more often in people who had severe COVID-19 illness, but anyone who has been infected with the virus that causes COVID-19 can experience post-COVID conditions. Research suggests that people who are vaccinated but experience a breakthrough infection are less likely to report post-COVID conditions, compared to people who are unvaccinated.

People with post-COVID conditions may develop or continue to have symptoms that are hard to explain and manage. Clinical evaluations and results of routine blood tests, chest x-rays, and electrocardiograms may be normal. The symptoms are similar to those reported by people with ME/CFS (myalgic encephalomyelitis/chronic fatigue syndrome) and other poorly understood chronic illnesses that may occur after other infections. Some people, especially those who had severe COVID-19, experience multiorgan effects or autoimmune conditions with symptoms lasting weeks, months, or even years after COVID-19 illness. Multi-organ effects can involve many body systems, including the brain, the kidneys, the liver, the lungs, the senses, the skin, the cardiovascular system, the endocrine system, the gastrointestinal system, the musculoskeletal system, and the nervous system. Post COVID conditions affect nearly every organ in the body and range from benign to life-threatening. As a result of these effects, people who have had COVID-19 may be more likely to develop new health conditions such as diabetes, heart conditions, blood clots, or neurological conditions compared with people who have not had COVID-19.

Conditions Affecting the Brain

People who recover from COVID-19 "exhibit significant cognitive deficits." These cognitive deficits include "brain fog . . .

low energy, difficulty concentrating, disorientation and difficulty finding the right words." Patients who were hospitalized and who received medical assistance for respiratory symptoms of COVID-19 developed greater cognitive deficits than patients who recovered at home. Cognitive deficits were greatest for patients who were put onto a ventilator but even patients with mild illness can experience cognitive deficits. One study found that fatigue and neurocognitive impairment are the two post-acute symptoms of COVID-19 that have the greatest impact on general health and working capacity for six to twelve months after recovering from acute COVID-19.

People who recover from COVID-19 experience a "reduction in grey matter thickness and tissue-contrast in the orbitofrontal cortex and parahippocampal gyrus . . . tissue damage in regions functionally-connected to the primary olfactory cortex and . . . reduction in global brain size." These effects were observed in both hospitalized and non-hospitalized patients and were associated with cognitive decline. Additional study is needed to determine whether these effects can be reversed over time.

Detailed data regarding the association between COVID-19 infection and sleep disorders is currently lacking. However, one study found that 26 percent of COVID-19 patients who were followed up after being discharged from the hospital reported sleep difficulties. Another study found that insomnia and sleep disturbances were commonly reported by patients recovering from COVID-19.

COVID-19 infection can cause the sudden worsening of a previous headache disorder, potentially making the headache disorder chronic. This is common with patients with migraine disorders. Some people without a history of migraine disorder have reported acquiring a migraine disorder as a result of a COVID-19 infection. Notably, some patients who did not experience headache during acute COVID-19 infection have developed persistent headaches following recovery from COVID-19. Symptoms of headache and migraine following recovery from COVID-19 are often closely associated with other symptoms of COVID-19, including insomnia, memory loss, dizziness, and fatigue, among others.

COVID-19 infection that reaches the brain can cause diverse neurological and dysexecutive syndromes, including aphasia, which is a language expression and comprehension disorder. Some patients experiencing acute COVID-19 infection have exhibited symptoms of aphasia, but the symptoms typically resolve within a few weeks to a few months following recovery from COVID-19. The incidence of aphasia in some patients can also be attributed to a stroke or blood clot caused by the acute COVID-19 infection.

One study found that, among patients diagnosed with COVID-19, 33 percent developed a neuropsychiatric disorder during the first six months of recovery. In the same period of time, nearly 13 percent of patients recovering from COVID-19 developed a neuropsychiatric disorder without having any prior history of such disorders. The risk for developing a neuropsychiatric disorder is greatest for patients who experienced severe COVID-19. The neuropsychiatric disorders studied include intracranial hemorrhage, ischemic stroke, Parkinsonism, Guillain-Barre syndrome, encephalitis, dementia, mood disorders, anxiety disorders, psychotic disorders, and substance use disorders, among others.

Conditions Affecting the Kidneys

One study found that people who recover from COVID-19 have an estimated 40 percent heightened risk of developing diabetes for up to a year following the initial infection. This risk exists even for people who had only mild symptoms of COVID-19 and the condition predominantly manifests as Type 2 Diabetes. Patients who were hospitalized or admitted to intensive care during their acute COVID-19 infection have roughly triple the risk of developing diabetes compared to people who did not have COVID-19. Another study found a significantly higher rate of new-onset diabetes in patients with COVID-19, which is associated with higher mortality rates and adverse events. A systematic and meta-analysis published in November 2022 found that COVID-19 survivors have a 66 percent increased chance of developing diabetes.

COVID-19 increases the risk of developing chronic kidney disease and acute kidney injury. Types of kidney damage include "inflammation, kidney fibrosis, and abnormal kidney gene expression." Patients who experienced severe COVID-19 are at the highest risk of developing these conditions. This risk endures for at least thirty days following a diagnosis with COVID-19. One study found that 35 percent of patients had reduced kidney function six months after recovering from COVID-19. Some patients may recover from kidney damage caused by COVID-19, but some damage to the kidneys caused by COVID-19 may be permanent. The long-term effects of COVID-19 on the kidneys are largely unknown.

Conditions Affecting the Liver

COVID-19 infection is associated with liver injury and liver-related complications. A series of post-mortem liver biopsies of COVID-19 patients revealed portal or sinusoidal vascular thrombosis in at least 50 percent of patients. Post-mortem findings suggest ischemic-type damage to the liver from COVID-19.

Patients with end-stage liver disease, including patients with cirrhosis who are decompensated, are at heightened risk of hospitalization, ventilation, and death from COVID-19.

Conditions Affecting the Lungs

People who recover from COVID-19 often experience persistent symptoms of lung damage, including pulmonary fibrosis. Pulmonary fibrosis is characterized by scarred lung tissue, decreased lung function, cough, and frailty. One study found that 20 percent of non-ventilated patients with COVID-19 displayed "fibrotic-like radiographic abnormalities" four months after hospitalization. The risk of pulmonary fibrosis is higher for patients with severe COVID-19 and those who received ventilator support during hospitalization. The damage to lung tissue caused by COVID-19 may be permanent.

Patients with asymptomatic or mild COVID-19 symptoms can develop lung abnormalities while patients who develop severe

COVID-19, characterized by viral pneumonia and respiratory failure, have a higher risk of developing persistent lung abnormalities. Symptoms of these abnormalities, including impaired lung function, persistent fatigue, decreased functional capacity and decreased quality of life, have been reported up to six months after hospital discharge.

Conditions Affecting the Senses

COVID-19 can cause damage to the eyes, including hemorrhages, cotton wool spots, retinal vein occlusions, arterial occlusions, localized retinal infarcts, and ocular inflammation. This damage can manifest between one and six weeks after the initial onset of COVID-19 symptoms.

One study found that COVID-19 can cause small nerve fibre damage in the cornea between four and twelve weeks after acute COVID-19 infection. This study found that the extent of corneal nerve damage is likely associated with the severity of COVID-19 infection.

Some people who have recovered from COVID-19 have reported sudden onset sensorineural hearing loss and tinnitus. One study found that patients with COVID-19 had "significantly worse high frequency pure tone audiometer thresholds and [transient evoked otoacoustic emissions] amplitudes," which suggests a potential relationship between COVID-19 infection and cochlear damage.

COVID-19 directly and indirectly acts on the nervous system, which can cause neuropathic pain. During acute COVID-19 infection, neuropathic pain manifests as "headache, dizziness, muscle pain, ataxia, and olfactory/taste disorders." One study found that neuropathic pain was reported by up to 2.3 percent of hospitalized COVID-19 patients, but suggested that the prevalence of neuropathic pain is underestimated because chronic neuropathic pain can arise months after injury to the nervous system. Neuropathic pain associated with COVID-19 can also be caused by acute ischemic stroke, acute transverse myelitis, and Guillain-Barre syndrome.

Conditions Affecting the Skin

Depending on the severity of a person's COVID-19 illness, they may develop one or more skin conditions. Asymptomatic disease can result in a Chilblain-like acral pattern, which typically affects the feet and hands and is associated with pain, burning, and itching. Mild COVID-19 can cause urticarial rash, which predominantly affects the trunk and limbs, with associated swelling. Mild COVID-19 can also cause confluent erythematous, maculopapular, or morbilliform rash, which are symmetrical lesions that start on the trunk and can cause itchiness from secondary lesions or skin eruptions. Papulovesicular exanthem is also associated with mild COVID-19, which is characterized either by small, widespread papules, vesicles, and pustules of varying sizes or a localized pattern of lesions on the chest, upper abdomen, or the back. COVID-19 can cause two ring-shaped lesions: mild COVID-19 can result in livedo reticularis-like lesions, which are transient, symmetrical, and dusky patches that form around a pale center; severe COVID-19 illness can result in livedo racemosa-like lesions, which are large, irregular, violet, and asymmetrical rings. Severe COVID-19 can also cause purpuric vasculitic pattern lesions, which affect peripheral body parts and regions where two skin areas meet or rub together. These lesions can evolve into hemorrhagic blisters and, ultimately, necrotic-ulcerative lesions. Fortunately, many of these skin conditions can be treated with topical corticosteroids and antihistamines.

Conditions Affecting the Cardiovascular System

Patients who recover from COVID-19 are at heightened risk of developing several cardiovascular conditions, including "abnormal heart rhythms, heart muscle inflammation, blood clots, strokes, myocardial infarction, and heart failure." Patients who experienced asymptomatic or mild COVID-19 illness are at risk of developing cardiovascular conditions as a consequence of the viral infection, but patients who were hospitalized had the highest risk of developing these conditions. One study found that these risks remained for twelve months following the initial COVID-19 infection.

Patients who recover from COVID-19 are at significantly higher risk for developing deep vein thrombosis, pulmonary embolism, and bleeding following the initial infection. The risk is highest for patients with severe illness caused by COVID-19 and one study observed a higher risk among patients who were exposed to COVID-19 during the first wave of the pandemic. The heightened risk of pulmonary embolism extended for up to six months after recovery from COVID-19, while the heightened risk for deep vein thrombosis extended for up to three months after recovery.

Up to six months after recovery from COVID-19, patients commonly experience chest pain, heart palpitations, and heartbeat irregularities. Patients with both mild and severe COVID-19 have a heightened risk of myocardial damage and myocarditis. One study found that the vascular system endures persistent inflammation following recovery from COVID-19, along with "significantly lower systemic vascular function and higher arterial stiffness." These patients were found to continue experiencing reduced cerebral vascular function and higher central arterial stiffness even if their other symptoms of COVID-19 had resolved. Additional research is needed to determine which cardiovascular complications will result in chronic illness.

Patients hospitalized for COVID-19 experience a higher risk of developing new-onset atrial fibrillation. One study found new-onset atrial fibrillation to be more common among patients who are white, male, older, and those who have pre-existing cardiovascular disease. This study found a 45.2 percent mortality rate for COVID-19 patients with new-onset atrial fibrillation.

A diagnosis with COVID-19 has a significant correlation with newly-onset erectile dysfunction in men. The cause for this relationship is not fully understood, but may be related to the location of ACE2 receptors in the testes, endothelial damage to erectile tissue, testicular damage, and psychological factors.

Conditions Affecting the Endocrine System

The coronavirus gains access to the human body through ACE2 receptors, which are found in several endocrine glands, including the pancreas, thyroid, ovaries, and testes. This makes the endocrine system vulnerable to destruction and alteration from COVID-19. Symptoms of damage to the endocrine system following COVID-19 infection include thyroid dysfunction, adrenal insufficiency, hypogonadism, changes to menstrual cycles, hyperglycemia, and ketoacidosis. Some of these symptoms can resolve on their own, but more research is needed to understand the long-term impacts that COVID-19 has on the endocrine system.

Conditions Affecting the Gastrointestinal System

The gastrointestinal system is vulnerable to damage from COVID-19 because it contains ACE2 receptors that the virus uses to access the body. Damage from COVID-19 can result in significant systemic disease involving the gastrointestinal tract, liver, biliary tract, and pancreas. Symptoms of damage to the gastrointestinal system include acute pancreatitis, anorexia, nausea, vomiting, diarrhea, gastrointestinal bleeding, lesions in the upper gastrointestinal tract, and ischemic lesions in the colon. One study found that COVID-19 patients sustained acute mucosal injuries to the gastrointestinal system and many had features of ischemic colitis, which is inflammation of the large intestine or colon.

Conditions Affecting the Musculoskeletal System

COVID-19 has widespread impacts on the musculoskeletal system, causing damage to the muscles, joints, nerves, soft tissues, and bone. Many patients report experiencing myalgia, which presents as muscle aches and pain, and myositis, which is muscle inflammation. Myositis can lead to rhabdomyolysis, which is a life-threatening condition associated with kidney failure, compartment syndrome, and intravascular coagulation. After recovering from COVID-19, patients may experience long-term symptoms of muscle damage, including sarcopenia (muscle loss) and cachexia (muscle wasting). Peripheral neuropathy, or nerve damage, is a common manifestation of COVID-19 illness. Peripheral neuropathy commonly manifests as pain, numbness, weakness, and tingling sensations. Guillain-Barre syndrome has also been reported, with symptoms beginning within three to four weeks after the initial onset of COVID-19 symptoms. This condition occurs as a result of nerve damage and causes muscle weakness and paralysis. COVID-19 has the ability to trigger rheumatological diseases, including "systemic lupus erythematosus, dermatomyositis, Graves' disease, rheumatoid arthritis, and psoriatic spondyloarthritis." The damage that COVID-19 causes to soft tissues can result in disseminated intravascular coagulation, gangrene, and bleeding complications.

One study examined how COVID-19 affected the skeletal system of mice and found that the virus caused significant decreases in bone volume and an increase in osteoclasts, which are cells that can lead to bone loss. Bone loss was observed even in mice who had asymptomatic COVID-19 infection. This study suggests that COVID-19 patients may be at a higher risk of developing osteoporosis and bone fractures, with the damage to the musculoskeletal system possibly being permanent.

Conditions Affecting the Nervous System

Some long-term symptoms of COVID-19 suggest that the virus damages the peripheral nervous system, which is responsible for signaling between the central nervous system and other parts of the body. Damage to this nervous system can manifest as difficulty coordinating muscle movements, muscle weakness and cramps, loss of senses, including taste, smell, touch, sight, and hearing, and interruption of regulatory functions, including breathing, digestion, heart, and gland functions. Symptoms of regulatory functions being interrupted include excessive or limited sweating, heat intolerance, blood pressure and heart rate irregularities, lightheadedness, and difficulty concentrating.

Fatigue is one of the most common symptoms that people experience after recovering from COVID-19. Researchers have observed many similarities between people who have recovered from COVID-19 and those who have myalgic encephalopathy and chronic fatigue syndrome. Symptoms of chronic fatigue can be linked to permanent damage that the virus causes to the heart, lungs, and the kidneys. Fatigue can also manifest as post-exertional malaise, which is the sudden onset of long-lasting extreme fatigue following ordinary activities. Many people overcome symptoms of chronic fatigue following recovery from COVID-19, but many others experience debilitating fatigue that does not improve.

Researchers have identified an association between COVID-19 and postural orthostatic tachycardia syndrome (POTS), which is a type of dysautonomia, or malfunction of the autonomic nervous system. This condition often manifests as inappropriate sinus tachycardia, where a patient experiences a higher heart rate response or resting heart rate than is necessary. Symptoms can also include chest pain, palpitations, and exercise intolerance. An estimated 2-14 percent of COVID-19 survivors are diagnosed with POTS, with 9-61 percent experiencing POTS-like symptoms.

The working definition of post-COVID conditions was developed by the Department of Health and Human Services (HHS) in collaboration with CDC and other partners. People who experience post-COVID conditions most commonly report; (https://www.cdc.gov/coronavirus/2019-ncov/long-term-effects/index.htm):

- Tiredness or fatigue that interferes with daily life.
- Symptoms that get worse after physical or mental effort (also known as "post-exertional malaise").
- Fever.
- Difficulty breathing or shortness of breath.

- Cough.

- Chest pain.

- Fast-beating or pounding heart (also known as heart palpitations).

- Difficulty thinking or concentrating (sometimes referred to as "brain fog").

- Headache.

- Sleep problems.

- Dizziness when you stand up (lightheadedness).

- Pins-and-needles feelings.

- Change in smell or taste.

- Depression or anxiety.

- Diarrhea.

- Stomach pain.

WHO also listed more "most common symptoms of post COVID-19 condition include:

- Fatigue

- Shortness of breath or difficulty breathing

- Memory, concentration or sleep problems

- Persistent cough

- Chest pain

- Trouble speaking

- Muscle aches

- Loss of smell or taste

- Depression or anxiety

- Fever

5.2 COST OF POST COVID

The long-terms symptoms of COVID-19 suggest that the virus damages or can damage multiple organs of human body. NIH and CDC are all conducting research to understand better the cost for long COVID. (https://www.aapmr.org/members-publications/covid-19/physiatrist-resource-center/long-covid-pasc-resources).

While the exact cause is not clear and is still under investigation, some evidence has suggested that symptoms and conditions could be related to one or more of the following (https://www.ruhealth.org/post-covid-treatment-options): chronic inflammation; small blood clots; dysregulation of the immune system; generation of auto-antibodies; organ damage; viral persistence; reactivation of other viruses (e.g., Epstein-Barr virus); sequelae of critical illness; exacerbations of underlying health conditions.

It is possible that even a person is tested negative, out of acute virus infection symptom, but a certain amount of virus still exists in the body. Through mutation, maybe the body's while cell do not kill them anymore. These remaining virus circulate through blood to the entire body organs, damaging any of these organs as times goes by, week, months, or years.

Another reason could be the leftover of cortisol which can affect every organ system in the body, (https://my.clevelandclinic.org/health/articles/22187-cortisol). Cortisol is a hormones that coordinate different functions in the body by carrying messages through your blood to your organs, skin, muscles and other tissues. It is an essential hormone that affects almost every organ and tissue in your body. cortisol can affect nearly every organ system in your body, including: nervous system; immune system; cardiovascular system; respiratory system; reproductive systems (female and male); musculoskeletal system; integumentary system (skin, hair, nails, glands and nerves). More specifically, cortisol affects your body by: regulating your body's stress response; regulating metabolism; suppressing inflammation; regulating blood pressure; increasing and regulating blood sugar; helping control your sleep-wake cycle.

Optimum cortisol levels are necessary for life and for maintaining several bodily functions. If you have consistently high or low cortisol levels, it can have negative impacts on your overall health. The level of cortisol in your blood, urine and saliva normally peaks in the early morning and declines throughout the day, reaching its lowest level around midnight. This pattern can change if you work a night shift and sleep at different times of the day. For most tests that measure cortisol levels in your blood, the normal ranges are:

- 6 a.m. to 8 a.m.: 10 to 20 micrograms per deciliter (mcg/dL).
- Around 4 p.m.: 3 to 10 mcg/dL.

5.3 POST COVID TREATMENT AND RECOVERY

In general, though, there are several everyday things you can do to try to lower your cortisol levels and keep them at optimal ranges, including:

Get quality sleep: Chronic sleep issues, such as obstructive sleep apnea, insomnia or working a night shift, are associated with higher cortisol levels.

Exercise regularly: Several studies have shown that regular exercise helps improve sleep quality and reduce stress, which can help lower cortisol levels over time.

Learn to limit stress and stressful thinking patterns: Being aware of your thinking pattern, breathing, heart rate and other signs of tension helps you recognize stress when it begins and can help you prevent it from becoming worse.

Practice deep breathing exercises: Controlled breathing helps stimulate your parasympathetic nervous system, your "rest and digest" system, which helps lower cortisol levels.

Enjoy yourself and laugh: Laughing promotes the release of endorphins and suppresses cortisol. Participating in hobbies and fun activities can also promote feelings of well-being, which may lower your cortisol levels.

Maintain healthy relationships: Relationships are a significant aspect of our lives. Having tense and unhealthy relationships with loved ones or coworkers can cause frequent stress and raise your cortisol levels.

It is very important to take care of your health, whether you've gotten the COVID-19 virus or not. These include to eat a balance and nutritious meal, to exercise regularly (walk, jogging, oxygen exercise is better), and sleeping well, etc. to allow the body heal and recover. Exercise need to be appropriate which make you feel good.

However, immediately after the symptom disappear, the body lost lots of cell, and is in the reproduction stage, so it is danger to do strong sports days after testing negative which can cause suddenly death.

People experiencing post-COVID conditions can seek care from a healthcare provider to come up with a personal medical management plan that can help improve their symptoms and quality of life. In addition, there are many support groups being organized that can help patients and their caregivers.

WHO stated that "At present, there is no specific medication therapy for people with post COVID-19 condition. However, there is data suggesting that holistic care, including rehabilitation, can be helpful."

Tollovid is a medicine for post-covid which went through clinical trial, but are not approved by the CDC, NIH or WHO yet.

TOLLOVID

Tollovid is a botanically – sourced commercial product that is available as a supplement and sold directly to consumers in the US and certain European markets, and has a Certificate of Free Sale. (https://mytollovid.com/pages/safety-toxicology-review).

Tollovid is delivered in capsule format and contains Lithospermum erythrorhizon (sometimes called Gromwell) root extract which demonstrates potent protease inhibitory activity, but is not supplemented with highly purified shikonin as is Tollovir. The recommended dose is 3 capsules 4 times daily for 5 days. Tollovid is developed by Todos Medical. It is sold for $149/bottle. (https://mytollovid.com/products/tollovid%E2%84%A2-immune-support-capsules).

REFERENCES

1 The Lancet Rheumatology 2 (7), e379-e381, 2020.

2. New England Journal of Medicine, 384 (1), 20-30, 2021.

3. International immunopharmacology 89, 107018, 2020.

4. Sobia Noreen, Irsah Maqbool, Asadullah Madni. European journal of pharmacology 894, 173854, 2021

5.   Dipayan Chaudhuri, Kiyoka Sasaki, Aram Karkar, Sameer Sharif, Kimberly Lewis, Manoj J Mammen, Paul Alexander, Zhikang Ye, Luis Enrique Colunga Lozano, Marie Warrer Munch, Anders Perner, Bin Du, Lawrence Mbuagbaw, Waleed Alhazzani, Stephen M Pastores, John Marshall, François Lamontagne, Djillali Annane, Gianfranco Umberto Meduri, Bram Rochwerg. Intensive care medicine 47 (5), 521-537, 2021

6. Jama 325 (7), 632-644, 2021.

7. Linda Gedded in Vaccines Work.

8. Raymond M Johnson, Joseph M Vinetz. Bmj 370, 2020.

9. The RECOVERY Collaborative Group. The New England journal of medicine, 2020

10. Journal of medical virology 92 (7), 814-818, 2020.

11. Journal of medical virology, 2020.

12. Journal of medical virology 92 (10), 2042-2049, 2020.

13. Journal of translational medicine 18 (1), 1-5, 2020.

14. La Rosèe et al., 2019.

15. Van der Ver et al., 2015.

16. International Journal of Infectious Diseases. Volume 96, July 2020, Pages 607-609.

17. The Lancet Rheumatology. Volume 2, Issue 7, July 2020, Pages e393-e400.

18. Sarah CJ Jorgensen, Christopher LY Tse, Lisa Burry, Linda D Dresser. Pharmacotherapy: The Journal of Human Pharmacology and Drug Therapy 40 (8), 843-856, 2020.

19. Infectious diseases and therapy 10 (4), 1933-1947, 202.

20. New England Journal of Medicine 385 (15), 1382-1392, 2021.

21. David M Weinreich, Sumathi Sivapalasingam, Thomas Norton, Shazia Ali, Haitao Gao, Rafia Bhore, Jing Xiao, Andrea T Hooper, Jennifer D Hamilton, Bret J Musser, Diana Rofail, Mohamed Hussein, Joseph Im, Dominique Y Atmodjo, Christina Perry, Cynthia Pan, Adnan Mahmood, Romana Hosain, John D Davis, Kenneth C

Turner, Alina Baum, Christos A Kyratsous, Yunji Kim, Amanda Cook, Wendy Kampman, Lilia Roque-Guerrero, Gerard Acloque, Hessam Aazami, Kevin Cannon, J Abraham Simón-Campos, Joseph A Bocchini, Bari Kowal, A Thomas DiCioccio, Yuhwen Soo, Gregory P Geba, Neil Stahl, Leah Lipsich, Ned Braunstein, Gary Herman, George D Yancopoulos. New England Journal of Medicine 385 (23), e81, 2021

22. Meagan P O'Brien, Eduardo Forleo-Neto, Bret J Musser, Flonza Isa, Kuo-Chen Chan, Neena Sarkar, Katharine J Bar, Ruanne V Barnabas, Dan H Barouch, Myron S Cohen, Christopher B Hurt, Dale R Burwen, Mary A Marovich, Peijie Hou, Ingeborg Heirman, John D Davis, Kenneth C Turner, Divya Ramesh, Adnan Mahmood, Andrea T Hooper, Jennifer D Hamilton, Yunji Kim, Lisa A Purcell, Alina Baum, Christos A Kyratsous, James Krainson, Richard Perez-Perez, Rizwana Mohseni, Bari Kowal, A Thomas DiCioccio, Neil Stahl, Leah Lipsich, Ned Braunstein, Gary Herman, George D Yancopoulos, David M Weinreich. New England Journal of Medicine 385 (13), 1184-1195, 2021.

23. Richard Copin, Alina Baum, Elzbieta Wloga, Kristen E Pascal, Stephanie Giordano, Benjamin O Fulton, Anbo Zhou, Nicole

Negron, Kathryn Lanza, Newton Chan, Angel Coppola, Joyce Chiu, Min Ni, Yi Wei, Gurinder S Atwal, Annabel Romero Hernandez, Kei Saotome, Yi Zhou, Matthew C Franklin, Andrea T Hooper, Shane McCarthy, Sara Hamon, Jennifer D Hamilton, Hilary M Staples, Kendra Alfson, Ricardo Carrion Jr, Shazia Ali, Thomas Norton, Selin Somersan-Karakaya, Sumathi Sivapalasingam, Gary A Herman, David M Weinreich, Leah Lipsich, Neil Stahl, Andrew J Murphy, George D Yancopoulos, Christos A Kyratsous. Cell 184 (15), 3949-3961. e11, 2021.

24. Samah Hayek, Yatir Ben-Shlomo, Noa Dagan, Ben Y Reis, Noam Barda, Eldad Kepten, Alina Roitman, Shachar Shapira, Shlomit Yaron, Ran D Balicer, Doron Netzer, Alon Peretz. Nature Communications 13 (1), 4480, 2022

25. George D Yancopoulos, David M Weinreich, Covid-19 Phase 2/3 Hospitalized Trial Team. medRxiv, 2021.11. 05.21265656, 2021

26. K Gary Barnette, Michael S Gordon, Domingo Rodriguez, T Gary Bird, Alan Skolnick, Michael Schnaus, Paula K Skarda, Suzana Lobo, Eduardo Sprinz, Georgi Arabadzhiev, Petar

Kalaydzhiev, Mitchell Steiner. NEJM Evidence 1 (9), EVIDoa2200145, 2022

27. Sylvia Rothenberger, Daniel L Hurdiss, Marcel Walser, Francesca Malvezzi, Jennifer Mayor, Sarah Ryter, Hector Moreno, Nicole Liechti, Andreas Bosshart, Chloe Iss, Valérie Calabro, Andreas Cornelius, Tanja Hospodarsch, Alexandra Neculcea, Thamar Looser, Anja Schlegel, Simon Fontaine, Denis Villemagne, Maria Paladino, Yvonne Kaufmann, Doris Schaible, Iris Schlegel, Dieter Schiegg, Christof Zitt, Gabriel Sigrist, Marcel Straumann, Julia Wolter, Marco Comby, Julia M Adler, Kathrin Eschke, Mariana Nascimento, Azza Abdelgawad, Achim D Gruber, Judith Bushe, Olivia Kershaw, Heyrhyoung Lyoo, Chunyan Wang, Wentao Li, Ieva Drulyte, Wenjuan Du, Kaspar Binz, Rachel Herrup, Sabrina Lusvarghi, Sabari Nath Neerukonda, Russell Vassell, Wei Wang, Susanne Mangold, Christian Reichen, Filip Radom, Charles G Knutson, Kamal K Balavenkatraman, Krishnan Ramanathan, Seth Lewis, Randall Watson, Micha A Haeuptle, Alexander Zürcher, Keith M Dawson, Daniel Steiner, Carol D Weiss, Patrick Amstutz, FJ van Kuppeveld, Michael T Stumpp, B Bosch, Olivier Engler, Jakob Trimpert.

28. Manon LM Prins, Johan L van der Plas, Maurits FJM Vissers, Cécile L Berends, Gaby Tresch, Marianne Soergel, Elena Fernández, Nikita van den Berge, Daniël Duijsings, Christof Zitt, Vaia Stavropoulou, Maya Zimmermann, Roxana F Drake, Jacobus Burggraaf, Geert H Groeneveld, Ingrid MC Kamerling. British Journal of Clinical Pharmacology, 2022.

29.   Luis Abrishamian, Marc Bonten, Richa Chandra, Damodaran Solai Elango, Pierre Fustier, Kinfemichael Gedif, Susana Goncalves, Awawu Igbinadolor, Jeff Kingsley, Charles G Knutson, Petra Kukkaro, Nagalingeswaran Kumarasamy, Philippe Legenne, Martha Mekebeb-Reuter, Krishnan Ramanathan, Evgeniya Reshetnyak, Michael Robinson, Jennifer Rosa, Marianne Soergel, Vaia Stavropoulou, Nina Stojcheva, Michael T Stumpp, Andreas Tietz, Xiaojun Zhao, Zhaojie Zhang. Open Forum Infectious Diseases 9 (Supplement 2), ofac492. 969, 2022.

30. Elisabeth Mahase. Bmj 372, 2021.

31. Humanities and Social Sciences Communications 9 (1), 1-12, 2022

32. Alex de Figueiredo, Clarissa Simas, Heidi J Larson.

33. Brobst B, Borger J.

34. Elizabeth C Lloyd, Tejal N Gandhi, Lindsay A Petty. JAMA 325 (10), 1015-1015, 2021.

35. Expert Opinion on Biological Therapy 22 (6), 763-780, 2022

36. Indian Journal of Anaesthesia 64 (10), 835, 2020

37. NM Allam, HM Eladl, MM Eid. Eur. Rev. Med. Pharmacol. Sci 15, 5618-5623, 2022.

38. Eye 34 (7), 1193-1195, 2020.

39. Medico-Legal Journal 88 (2), 76-77, 2020.

40. New England Journal of Medicine 382 (18), 1679-1681, 2020).

41. Public Money & Management 40 (6), 483-485, 2020

42. The American journal of gastroenterology, 2020.

43. The Journal of the American Board of Family Medicine 34 (Supplement), S61-S70, 2021.

44. Nature Reviews Nephrology volume 19, pages 38–52 (2023).

45. Torres A, et al. Effect of corticosteroids on treatment failure among hospitalized patients with severe community-acquired

pneumonia and high inflammatory response: A randomized clinical trial. JAMA. 2015;313:677.

46. Keller MJ, et al. Effect of systemic glucocorticoids on mortality or mechanical ventilation in patients with COVID-19. Journal of Hospital Medicine. 2020;15:489.

47. Odeyemi YE, et al. Early, biomarker-guided steroid dosing in COVID-19 pneumonia: A pilot randomized controlled trial. Critical Care. 2022;26:9.

48. Centers for Disease Control and Prevention. Pneumonia.

49. World Health Organization. COVID-19 China.

50. American Lung Association. Acute respiratory distress syndrome (ARDS).

51. Grant RA, Morales-Nebreda L, Markov NS, et al. Circuits between infected macrophages and T cells in SARS-CoV-2 pneumonia. *Nature*. 2021;590(7847):635-641. doi:10.1038/s41586-020-03148-w

52. Zhao D, Yao F, Wang L, et al. A comparative study on the clinical features of coronavirus 2019 (COVID-19) pneumonia with other pneumonias. *Clinical Infectious Diseases*. 2020;71(15):756-761. doi:10.1093/cid/ciaa247

53. Centers for Disease Control and Prevention. Symptoms of COVID-19.

54. Centers for Disease Control and Prevention. COVID-19 treatments and medications.

55. COVID-19 Treatment Guidelines Panel. Coronavirus Disease 2019 (COVID-19) Treatment Guidelines. National Institutes of Health. Available at https://www.covid19treatmentguidelines.nih.gov/ Accessed 1/23/2023.

56. Centers for Disease Control and Prevention. SARS-CoV-2 variant classifications and definitions. 2022. Available at: https://www.cdc.gov/coronavirus/2019-ncov/variants/variant-classifications.html. Accessed August 16, 2022.

57. Food and Drug Administration. Fact sheet for healthcare providers: Emergency Use Authorization for Evusheld (tixagevimab co-packaged with cilgavimab). 2022. Available at: https://www.fda.gov/media/154701/ download.

58. Cameroni E, Bowen JE, Rosen LE, et al. Broadly neutralizing antibodies overcome SARS-CoV-2 Omicron antigenic

shift. Nature. 2022;602(7898):664-670. Available at: https://www.ncbi.nlm.nih.gov/pubmed/35016195.

59. Liu L, Iketani S, Guo Y, et al. Striking antibody evasion manifested by the Omicron variant of SARS-CoV-2. Nature. 2022. Available at: https://www.ncbi.nlm.nih.gov/pubmed/35016198.

OTHER REFERENCES

1. New England Journal of Medicine 384 (1), 20-30, 2021

2. Mino-León D, Galván-Plata ME, Doubova SV, Flores-Hernandez S, Reyes-Morales H. A pharmacoepidemiological study of potential drug interactions and their determinant factors in hospitalized patients. Rev Invest Clin 2011; 63:170–178. [PubMed] [Google Scholar]

3. Alvim MM, Silva LA, Leite IC, Silvério MS. Adverse events caused by potential drug-drug interactions in an intensive care unit of a teaching hospital. Rev Bras Ter Intensiva 2015; 27:353–359. doi: 10.5935/0103-507X.20150060 [PMC free article] [PubMed] [Google Scholar].

4. Moura C, Prado N, Acurcio F. Potential drug-drug interactions associated with prolonged stays in the intensive

care unit: a retrospective cohort study. Clin Drug Investig 2011; 31:309–316. Doi: 10.2165/11586200-000000000-00000 [PubMed] [Google Scholar].

WEBSITE REFERENCE:

1. https://icmanaesthesiacovid-19.org/background#:~:text=The%20virus%20causing%20the%20infection,airborne%20High%20Consequence%20Infections%20Disease

2. https://www.un.org/en/coronavirus/covid-19-faqs

3. https://www.who.int/news-room/questions-and-answers/item/coronavirus-disease-covid-19-dexamethasone#:~:text=Dexamethasone%20is%20a%20corticosteroid%20used,benefits%20for%20critically%20ill%20patients

4. https://www.who.int/news/item/22-04-2022-who-recommends-highly-successful-covid-19-therapy-and-calls-for-wide-geographical-distribution-and-transparency-from-originator

5. https://www.gavi.org/vaccineswork/everything-you-need-know-about-covid-19-antivirals

6. https://www.covid19treatmentguidelines.nih.gov/therapies/antivirals-including-antibody-products/remdesivir/#:~:text=In%20nonhospitalized%20patients%20with%20mild,hospital%20discharge%2C%20whichever%20comes%20first

7. https://www.who.int/news-room/questions-and-answers/item/coronavirus-disease-(covid-19)-vaccines-safety

8. https://www.who.int/news/item/16-04-2021-global-advisory-committee-on-vaccine-safety-(gacvs)-review-of-latest-evidence-of-rare-adverse-blood-coagulation-events-with-astrazeneca-covid-19-vaccine-(vaxzevria-and-covishield)

9. https://www.who.int/news/item/19-05-2021-statement-gacvs-safety-johnson-johnson-janssen-covid-19-vaccine

10. https://www.who.int/news/item/26-07-2021-statement-of-the-who-gacvs-covid-19-subcommittee-on-gbs

11. https://www.mayoclinic.org/diseases-conditions/coronavirus/in-depth/coronavirus-long-term-effects/art-20490351

12. https://health-desk.org/articles/what-short-and-long-term-effects-does-covid-19-have-on-other-body-parts-including-lungs-brain-heart-and-kidneys

13. https://www.nhs.uk/conditions/coronavirus-covid-19/self-care-and-treatments-for-coronavirus/how-to-treat-symptoms-at-home/

14. https://www.mayoclinic.org/diseases-conditions/coronavirus/diagnosis-treatment/drc-20479976

15. https://www.ncbi.nlm.nih.gov/pmc/articles/PMC5755936/#ref-list-1title

16. https://vaccination-info.eu/en/vaccination/benefits-vaccination-community

17. https://www.sciencedirect.com/science/article/pii/S2665991320301648

18. https://www.sciencedirect.com/science/article/pii/S1201971220303337

19. https://medlineplus.gov/druginfo/meds/a602001.html#:~:text=Anakinra%20is%20authorized%20for%20the,adds%20oxygen%20to%20the%20blood

20. https://my.clevelandclinic.org/health/treatments/22246-monoclonal-antibodies

21. https://www.mayoclinic.org/drugs-supplements/baricitinib-oral-route/side-effects/drg-20487070

22. https://www.mskcc.org/cancer-care/patient-education/medications/bamlanivimab-and-etesevimab#:~:text=Tell%20your%20doctor%20right%20away%20if%20you%20have%20fever%20or,lips%2C%20face%2C%20or%20throat%3B

23. https://www.clinicalstudydatarequest.com/

24. https://www.who.int/news-room/feature-stories/detail/the-novavax-vaccine-against-covid-19-what-you-need-to-know

25. https://www.reuters.com/business/healthcare-pharmaceuticals/who-issues-emergency-use-listing-novavax-serum-institutes-covid-19-vaccine-2021-12-17/

26. https://www.gov.uk/government/publications/regulatory-approval-of-covid-19-vaccine-nuvaxovid

27. https://www.tga.gov.au/resources/auspmd/nuvaxovid

28. https://www.ema.europa.eu/en/news/ema-starts-rolling-review-novavaxs-covid-19-vaccine-nvx-cov2373

29. https://www.nps.org.au/australian-prescriber/articles/sars-cov-2-rs-nvx-cov-2373-vaccine-for-prevention-of-covid-19

30. https://www.who.int/news-room/feature-stories/detail/who-can-take-the-pfizer-biontech-covid-19--vaccine-what-you-need-to-know

31. https://www.cdc.gov/coronavirus/2019-ncov/vaccines/expect/after.html

32. https://www.fda.gov/emergency-preparedness-and-response/coronavirus-disease-2019-covid-19/moderna-covid-19-vaccines

33. https://www.who.int/news-room/feature-stories/detail/the-moderna-covid-19-mrna-1273-vaccine-what-you-need-to-know

34. https://www.cdc.gov/vaccines/covid-19/info-by-product/moderna/reactogenicity.html

35.   https://www.medicalnewstoday.com/articles/how-long-do-side-effects-of-moderna-vaccine-last#first-and-second-dose-side-effects

36.   https://www.medicalnewstoday.com/articles/how-long-do-side-effects-of-moderna-vaccine-last#vs-other-vaccines

37.   https://www.eatthis.com/best-foods-fight-covid-symptoms/?utm_source=msn&utm_medium=feed&utm_campaign=msn-feed

38.   https://publichealth.jhu.edu/2021/use-of-dexamethasone-remdesivir-against-covid-19-varied-widely-across-us-health-systems

39.   https://www.cdc.gov/coronavirus/2019-ncov/your-health/treatments-for-severe-illness.html

40.   https://www.yalemedicine.org/news/9-things-to-know-about-covid

pill#:~:text=Molnupiravir%20is%20authorized%20for%20the,affect%20bone%20and%20cartilage%20growth

41.   https://m.timesofindia.com/life-style/health-fitness/health-news/coronavirus-using-oxygen-at-home-here-are-some-dos-and-donts-to-follow/amp_etphotostory/82309021.cms

42.	https://www.cdc.gov/coronavirus/2019-ncov/global-covid-19/telemedicine.html

43.	https://www.yalemedicine.org/news/13-things-to-know-paxlovid-covid-19

44.	https://www.mayoclinic.org/tests-procedures/convalescent-plasma-therapy/about/pac-20486440

45.	https://www.goodrx.com/conditions/covid-19/coronavirus-treatments-on-the-way

46.	https://www.goodrx.com/conditions/covid-19/covid-19-boosters

47.	https://www.who.int/news-room/questions-and-answers/item/coronavirus-disease-covid-19-dexamethasone

48.	https://www.eatthis.com/best-foods-fight-covid-symptoms/?utm_source=msn&utm_medium=feed&utm_campaign=msn-feed

49.	https://www.nhs.uk/medicines/molnupiravir/side-effects-of-molnupiravir/

50.	https://www.mayoclinic.org/drugs-supplements/sarilumab-subcutaneous-route/side-effects/drg-20406298

51. World Health Organization. Tracking SARS-CoV-2 variants. 2022. Available at: https://www.who.int/en/activities/tracking-SARS-CoV-2-variants.

52. Post COVID Resource: https://www.aapmr.org/members-publications/covid-19/physiatrist-resource-center/long-covid-pasc-resources

53. Post-COVID https://pandemicpatients.org/home/covid-19-resources/post-covid-conditions/?gclid=Cj0KCQiAw8OeBhCeARIsAGxWtUwVx8wReWsr9dXUSrp9MFxDVmj_w1RyfbPMZzvGZHufvqE3-ngEQO8aAhqOEALw_wcB

ABOUT THE AUTHOR

Susan Su holds a Ph.D. from U. C. Berkeley in engineering. She worked in the National Berkeley National Lab, consulted for NASA--National Aeronautics and Space Administration. She published many scientific papers at international and national journals.